# PRACTICING HARM REDUCTION PSYCHOTHERAPY

# *Practicing Harm Reduction Psychotherapy*

## An Alternative Approach to Addictions

**Patt Denning**

*Foreword by G. Alan Marlatt*

THE GUILFORD PRESS
New York London

© 2000 Patt Denning

Published by The Guilford Press

A Division of Guilford Publications, Inc.

72 Spring Street, New York, NY 10012

www.guilford.com

Printed in the United States of America

This book is printed on acid-free paper.

Last digit is print number:   9   8   7   6   5   4   3   2   1

Library of Congress Cataloging-in-Publication Data is available from the Publisher.

ISBN 1-57230-555-X

# *About the Author*

**Patt Denning, PhD,** has been working in the field of mental health and substance abuse for 25 years. She is dedicated to the development of alternative perspectives and treatment models that can address the complex needs of patients presenting with multiple problems. Dr. Denning worked as a director of both residential and outpatient psychiatric programs for the San Francisco Division of Mental Health for 16 years. In her private practice she focuses not only on individual treatment, but also on staff training and development in the area of harm reduction. In 1997, she earned a diplomate in psychopharmacology. A past core faculty member of the San Francisco School of Psychology, Dr. Denning is currently an adjunct faculty member at the American School of Psychology, Richmond, California, campus. She is also a media expert for the Partnership for Responsible Drug Information.

# *Acknowledgments*

Many people have helped me launch and finish this book. (Sometimes it felt more like a conspiracy than a support group!) Nevertheless, I have many people to thank and no one but myself to accept responsibility for the final product.

I would never have undertaken this project without the firm encouragement and brutal arm twisting of Pat Sax and the unconditional support of G. Alan Marlatt. I would not have completed it without the constant efforts of my partner and editorial assistant, Kathie Cinnater, who spent many hours editing the drafts and providing comic relief, emotional support, hot meals, and clean laundry.

Kathy Chavez, Amy Wilner, Virginia Crowder, and David Steinberg provided much needed editorial review.

Of course, my patients, students, and colleagues helped me formulate my ideas and provided important details that enrich the various sections. Special thanks to Edith Springer and Sara Kershner from the Harm Reduction Coalition, who gave support from afar.

I am also thankful to a select group of friends/colleagues who, during the final stages of writing, formed a harm reduction *salon*—reading the manuscript and meeting en masse to give me feedback: Peter Goetz, Peter Goldblum, Sally Hand, Alesia Kunz, Jeannie Little, Kevin McGirr, Helen Marlo, Lisa Moore, Liz Naidoff, and Michael Siever.

Finally, I am indebted to the many men and women who have come to me with their alcohol and drug problems. They are the originators and the primary beneficiaries of this work.

# Foreword

*I*t gives me considerable pleasure to introduce Patt Denning's *Practicing Harm Reduction Psychotherapy: An Alternative Approach to Addictions*, to my knowledge, the first book to provide a comprehensive overview of this unique and still emerging approach to the treatment of addictive behavior problems. This excellent book is written for psychotherapists by a therapist who herself has developed considerable clinical experience in applying this model in the clinical setting.

I first met Patt at a harm reduction conference held a few years ago. At the conference, a small group of psychotherapists, including Patt, Andrew Tatarsky, myself, and a few other colleagues, convened for the first time to discuss applications of the harm reduction model in the treatment of clients with active, ongoing addictive behaviors such as harmful drinking or drug use. The possibility of developing an integrative harm reduction approach in the treatment of co-occurring disorders such as alcohol dependence and depression was also discussed. Overall, it was an exciting, ground-breaking meeting as we came to the realization that harm reduction methods, originally designed to reduce the harmful consequences of ongoing drug use (e.g., needle exchange for active heroin users), could provide a bridge to cross the "great disconnect" that exists between the substance abuse and mental health treatment fields. Although the problem of how to treat people with a "dual diagnosis" of both substance abuse and a psychiatric disorder has been raised by providers on both sides of the fence, this dispute appeared to us to be rooted in a professional controversy about which of the two disciplines had primary "owner-ship" for the treatment of these clients. Thus the issue of dual diag-nosis became one of "dueling diagnostics" fueled largely by a turf war over who would receive funding for providing treatment ser-vices. The advent of managed care, and the push toward developing a unified treatment approach for what have come to be called "behavioral health" problems, provided further impetus for integrat-ing intervention programs for clients with co-occurring disorders.

This book provides a blueprint for therapists who wish to pro-vide such an integrated approach to the treatment of a variety of addictive behaviors, with or without the co-occurrence of other psy-chological or behavioral disorders. For the first time, clients who wish to receive therapy to help them cope with an ongoing alcohol or other drug problem will not be turned away at the door either by substance abuse counselors (who insist upon abstinence as the only acceptable treatment goal) or by mental health therapists (who often refer active drug users to substance abuse treatment before they will accept them for psychotherapy). Many clients, particularly those with co-occurring disorders, are confused and discouraged by this professional debate.

To take one example, I recently interviewed a woman who had dual problems with alcohol and depression. During the conversation, she mentioned that she felt puzzled and confused about what she had been told previously by other therapists she had consulted. She first contacted a psychiatrist, who told her that her drinking problems were caused by her depression, and that her attempts to "self-medicate" depressive symptoms with alcohol would put her at risk for alcohol dependence. This psychiatrist refused to treat her for depression unless she first committed herself to an alcoholism treat-ment program. When she then visited an alcoholism treatment coun-selor, she was told that her drinking problem was the primary cause of her depression, and that if she gave up alcohol, her depression would be alleviated. The counselor told her that she needed residen-tial treatment for her primary disease of alcoholism and recom-mended against any concurrent treatment for her depression (espe-cially the use of antidepressant medications). No wonder she felt confused. I asked her, "What do you think is true—that your alcohol problems are caused by your depression or that your depression is caused by drinking?" After a thoughtful pause, she replied, "For me, the truth is somewhere in the middle. My drinking and my depression seem to be linked together in a reciprocal kind of way. Sometimes I drink to forget things when I feel depressed. At other times, however, such as after a bout of drinking, I often feel depressed and guilty about what I did."

I agreed to work with this woman and to provide an integrated harm reduction approach to working with both her alcohol and depression problems. Over several months of treatment, she developed a deeper understanding of the reciprocal nature of her negative mood swings and excessive drinking episodes. At first she selected a goal of moderate drinking, saying that she was afraid to give up alcohol altogether because drinking was her main way of coping. As she learned other ways to manage her depression (meditation and marital therapy were particularly helpful for her), she eventually elected to abstain from alcohol. At this point, the goal of harm reduction therapy was linked to a relapse prevention approach as we worked together to manage her occasional lapses to drinking during the next several months. At the completion of therapy, she had attained her goal of stable abstinence and was making considerable progress in managing her depressive episodes. By following her priorities (instead of my insisting upon abstinence as an initial requirement for treatment), she successfully made the transition from harmful drinking to abstinence. "If abstinence was required as a precondition for me to get any therapy at the beginning," she told me, "I would never have started treatment of any kind."

Harm reduction therapy, as illustrated throughout this book, provides a client-centered approach to working with people "where they are" rather than "where they should be" as dictated by treatment providers. By allowing clients to set their own goals and to continue to provide support and assistance as their goals change over time, harm reduction therapy is consumer oriented, its focus on informed choice and a partnership approach between therapist and client. This focus on consumer choice makes harm reduction therapy "user friendly" for active drug users who seek therapy and reduces the stigma associated with traditional alcohol or drug treatment programs. It embodies the "low-threshold" principle of harm reduction, in which traditional barriers to treatment seeking are removed, including insisting upon initial commitment to abstinence as the only acceptable goal. Research has shown that harm reduction programs are more likely to attract active drug users, to motivate them to begin to make changes in their behavior, to retain these individuals longer in treatment, and to minimize attrition and dropout rates. By embracing a comprehensive biopsychosocial model of addictive behavior, harm reduction therapy is more likely than a traditional biological disease model to enhance client self-efficacy and motivation for change. From the harm reduction perspective, addictive habits can be changed, one step at a time. Habit change is often an incremental process, and any positive change in terms of reducing harmful consequences is considered a "step in the right direction."

Patt Denning represents many of the qualities that I believe characterize a successful harm reduction therapist. In reading through these chapters, I was impressed time and time again by these qualities. First, Patt comes across as a warm and empathic therapist. In her case study presentations, her humanistic approach is clearly revealed by her nonjudgmental and accepting clinical approach. At the same time, her clinical work is solidly based in pragmatism rather than on moral idealism—Patt is more interested in coming up with clinical strategies that work, as compared to following rigid moral ideologies. Her clinical stance is open-minded, and she is more than willing to challenge the existing rigid orthodoxy of the predominant disease model of addiction. In short, Patt Denning's work illustrates the breadth and talent that make an ideal therapist in the harm reduction field. At the same time, it is important to note that her exemplary qualities are often the same ones we all associate with good psychotherapists in general, no matter what type of clinical problems they work with. And this point emerges as one of the central messages of this book: that it is finally time to bring the basic principles of psychotherapy back into the treatment of addictive behaviors. Patt Denning provides a trail-blazing journey into the new world of harm reduction therapy. I hope readers enjoy and benefit from this book as much as I did!

G. ALAN MARLATT, PHD
*University of Washington*

# Preface

*I*t is no longer possible to be a psychotherapist and work only with people who have emotional problems uncomplicated by the use of intoxicating substances. Despite the fact that my education provided very little explicit training in drug and alcohol problems, I encountered many patients for whom depression, anxiety, or psychosis was intertwined with the use or abuse of drugs. After finding traditional chemical dependency theory and treatment limited for these patients, primarily because of the complex interaction of drugs and mental disorders, I set out to discover other approaches. Thus began a long process of developing my own way of working with these complex issues.

This book is the result of a professional journey through several fields of interest. The most recent, and most useful, is a public health model called harm reduction (or risk reduction in some other countries). Its philosophy is simple; yet, with it, I was able to conceptualize complex problems and develop alternative treatment methods to work with people with drug or alcohol problems. This book presents my model of what is being termed *harm reduction psychotherapy*. It is based on the belief that addictions are biopsychosocial phenomena and can best be treated with a complex and integrated form of psychotherapy.

Learning to abide by the principles of harm reduction was the end result of traveling many professional roads. The first task of my early career was to create and teach a program of drug, alcohol, and sex education in a maximum security juvenile center. I ended my work as a special education teacher when I completed a master's degree in Counseling Psychology. For the next 15 years, I worked in community mental health settings as a director, supervisor, and direct service clinician. I had little training in drug or alcohol problems other than a course in psychopharmacology during my doctoral program. This gap in knowledge was not overly problematic, however, because at that time, the community mental health system attempted to make a rigorous distinction between people with mental health problems and those who were "addicts and alcoholics."

Beginning in 1983, however, I worked as the director of a large outpatient psychiatric program that was part of a primary care public health service located in a predominantly gay and lesbian area of San Francisco. The new HIV epidemic was causing traumatic losses and fear in the community, and both mental health problems and substance use were increasing. The extreme stress and anxiety of the situation brought together the medical, nursing, and mental health staff in a way that was unusual. We shared information, fears, and encouragement as we developed state-of-the-art interventions to help those who had fallen ill. As a staff committed to community work, we sometimes tried to include attention to substance abuse as part of our regular psychiatric treatment in order not to split the treatment of our fragile patients. More often, however, we facilitated referral to a drug treatment program. It was during the course of discussions with staff at these programs, and attendance at some of their trainings and 12-Step meetings, that I first learned about the disease model and the nature of addiction and recovery.

Even with this exposure, I was not entirely sure how to apply the concepts of disease model treatment to the psychodynamic work I was doing. Just as important, I did not really believe in many of the "truths" that I was being told. It was hard for me to believe that addictions are diseases or that they always progress toward extreme consequences. Nevertheless, I had no other solid basis on which to conduct treatment, so I deferred to the expertise of chemical dependency counselors. Most patients who had drug problems were referred out for treatment, but many of the most psychologically fragile patients stayed in our clinic for treatment by the mental health staff. By the end of 1990, at least half of our patients were dually diagnosed, and many of them suffered from HIV infection as well.

The cases I present in Chapter 1 are examples of the difficulties I encountered trying to use disease model and 12-Step methods in my work. In each case, my therapeutic interventions caused more harm to my patients than did the drugs they were using. These cases haunted me for a long time. I began to realize that while many of my patients' problems were obviously affected by their use of substances, they generally had other, psychological, issues. It occurred to me that the distinction between mental health and substance abuse theory and treatment was not as clear as practitioners suggested, but I had few professional resources to help me clarify a new position. Since I had received some training in psychopharmacology, I was not altogether ignorant of the physiological effects of drugs, but I lacked formal training in chemical dependency and was naive about the nature of the relationship that exists between the user and the drug of choice. Over a relatively short period of time, I realized that, despite my efforts, patients were dropping out of treatment or not getting better. I became convinced that traditional chemical dependency notions of assessment and treatment were too simplistic and not sufficiently individualized. I began to look again at traditional ways of working with drug use problems and attempted to rethink some ideas and reconcile often-competing mental health principles. The following case sheds some light on my dilemmas.

Kate presented me with assessment and treatment dilemmas that were beyond the scope of my expertise at the time. She was HIV positive, probably as a result of intravenous speed use. While she was asymptomatic medically, she was extremely anxious and depressed, complaining of lethargy and of having an "old brain" because she could not concentrate as well as usual. She was struggling with her drug use on her own because she feared losing her job if her employer found out. We had little guidance to develop a treatment plan for such a client, so I referred her to drug treatment as an initial step, thinking that we could focus on other issues once she had become clean and sober. It did not occur to me, or to others on the treatment team, to evaluate her cognitive symptoms for evidence of HIV dementia, or to take her complaints of depression and anxiety seriously from a psychiatric perspective. Speed can cause both anxiety and depression, and we assumed that abstinence would significantly alter her presentation.

When she failed to follow up on the referral to drug treatment, I was concerned, but decided that she just was not "ready for treatment." She returned a year later, still using speed, still anxious and depressed, and unemployed and homeless. While one could blame the drug use on this negative outcome, I asked her opinion about what had happened. I was shocked when she expressed both anger at me and self-hatred. She took my referral as a way to "dump" her because she was too needy and "messed-up." Unaccustomed to asserting herself, she escaped back into her self-destructive lifestyle until her physical health deteriorated. Even though one might argue that she had not yet "hit bottom" a year earlier and only now was ready for treatment, I concluded that the amount of harm that had accrued to her in that time was unacceptable to me as a therapist. Why did I think that drug users were any different from other patients with purely emotional problems? And why did I suggest that she try to fix only one aspect of her life, with no attention to other pressing problems?

Cases such as Kate's recurred over the years and I became determined to find other ways of conceptualizing patients' drug use. I had some success and much frustration. The therapeutic technique of confrontation rather than exploration seemed hurtful and bound to increase resistance. My patients and I struggled with their problems, and many of them did not get better. As I began to study both psychotherapy and chemical dependency treatment models, I found it extremely difficult to integrate them, and realized that limitations in each were hard to overcome.

I grew increasingly resistant to some of the tenets of 12-Step-based interventions, particularly the emphasis on powerlessness and spirituality. I also became aware that traditional disease model approaches are ineffective for many drug users, resulting in a revolving door comprised of short-term abstinence and relapses. But despite a low success rate, there has been little development of new approaches and little disagreement allowed within such programs. The people I spoke with in the chemical dependency field assured me that most addicts do not "make it," and that I needed to accept this fact and not be so "overinvolved" with my patients.

The limitations of psychological theories and practices became obvious to me as well. In the field of chemical dependency, psychotherapists have opted out of important debates regarding causation and best treatment strategies. Indeed, standard psychotherapeutic approaches have had little success with drug users. Several factors are at play. Adaptive models generally view drug use patterns only as symptoms of underlying problems or as indications of skills deficits. Additionally, most psychotherapists lack sufficient training to conduct a drug use history and miss information essential to treatment planning. Some mental health professionals consider the psychopathology of these patients too severe to treat because they feel most addicts are impulse-ridden people with sociopathic personality disorders. The added burden of addiction made any of my efforts seem wasted. Perhaps, suggested some mental health professionals, I should look at why I could not accept the wisdom of the clinicians in either the field of chemical dependency or the field of psychotherapy. It seemed that few shared my discomfort with the treatment of these patients.

There are, however, several cognitive and behavioral approaches specifically designed for alcohol and drug problems. This literature, which was unknown to me at the time, opened up therapeutic possibilities once I found it. Specific techniques such as desensitization, identification of high-risk situations for drug use, and drink refusal training offer exciting possibilities for real change. These models did not, however, contribute to my belief in developmental processes such as affect tolerance and unconscious defenses. Cognitive-behavioral approaches, which seemed excellent in terms of technique, lacked the needed complexity to work effectively with people whose serious drug problems were intertwined with mental disorders.

Caught between two strong belief systems, and feeling alone, I decided to use traditional psychodynamic principles as a guide. I studied the impact of defenses and attempted to work on the premise that substance abuse is symptomatic of underlying psychopathology. It became apparent that by doing this, I was ignoring the very real effects of drugs on the patient. I saw the similarities between the concept of transferred addictions (when a person quits one drug and eventually becomes addicted to something else) and the psychodynamic work on symptom substitution but could not bridge the theoretical gap between them. But when I added a little bit of 12-Step theory to the therapeutic mix, I realized that I could not say that drug addiction was both a symptom of some other primary problem and a primary disease in and of itself.

In discovering that my own efforts to synthesize treatment methods were not working, I hoped for some open discussion with my colleagues in chemical dependency treatment settings. I learned, however, that professionals from the chemical dependency field and the mental health field are often quite critical of each other, with relationships marked by either a lack of communication or animosity. There was very little sharing of perspectives to help me develop a coherent approach. In trying to combine techniques from these models, I was actually straddling paradigms, those conceptual territories whose inhabitants are often fiercely protective of their professional space. My attempt to shift paradigms and develop a different way of looking at substance use problems led me toward developing an addiction treatment that stood apart from traditional notions and allowed the exploration of different approaches. I quickly learned that many people were interested in just such an option.

At the time, I did not recognize that much of what I was thinking about the changes needed in substance use treatment had a foundation in the public health movement in the United States and abroad. Since I was working in just such a setting, I used it as an opportunity to see how a community-based, public health model might inform a mental health treatment model. I thank the staff of San Francisco's Health Center # 1 for their support and guidance as I discovered the harm reduction movement and brought it into traditional psychiatric treatment to form an integrated treatment for people with substance use disorders.

In 1994, I discovered a new organization, the Harm Reduction Coalition, and realized that its philosophy could bridge the gap between public health approaches and direct clinical applications. An important aspect of harm reduction is its sociopolitical analysis of drug problems and of the therapeutic interventions that have arisen from the conservative agenda that rules in this country. Drug use exists within a matrix of individuals, social and political systems, and cultural beliefs. It has even become an integral part of subculture or racial identity in certain groups. Our response in the United States has been one of fear, coercive treatments, and punitive measures. One cannot ignore this reality or remove a sociopolitical perspective from any drug and alcohol treatment approach without turning it into just another in a series of techniques to be applied in uniform settings without attendance to individual differences. The practice of harm reduction requires a significant shift in perspective, one that allows that the client is, in fact, a consumer requesting assistance with self-defined problems. This "bottom up" (Marlatt, 1998) flow of power in the therapeutic relationship is an essential part of what we call harm reduction psychotherapy. This treatment paradigm demands that the therapist respect the choices a person might make and offer help when these choices result in harm, without demanding that the client make changes that only the therapist (or society) wants.

The harm reduction movement, being consumer led, is sensitive to the subtle prejudices that linger in even the most earnest person. The use of pejorative language is a central criticism directed at health care providers. In writing this book, I examined my attitudes, biases, and language many times. Chapter 1 has a section on the meaning and use of certain terms in the addiction field. The following section, however, is a strictly personal account of my own struggle with the words "patient" and "client."

## THE LANGUAGE OF CLINICIANS: A PERSONAL ACCOUNT

It is often possible to identify the specific discipline of individuals based on their use of the term "patient" versus "client" to describe people who come for help. Most drug treatment workers refer to program members as either participants or clients. Staff of residential programs in both drug treatment and some psychiatric treatment settings often use the term "resident" to describe program participants, wishing to emphasize the fact that they are creating a home for themselves within the treatment program. Medical personnel routinely use the word "patient." Mental health providers seem the most inconsistent in their reference to people who come to them for therapy. Using the word "patient" underscores the assumed nature of the relationship as one of sufferer and healer, sick and healthy. (The original meaning of "patient" is "one who suffers.") It is not a far stretch, psychologically speaking, from "sick and healthy" to "bad and good," or certainly, "powerless and powerful." On the other hand, the word "client," while emphasizing the consumer aspects of the helping relationship, tends to downplay the power imbalance that often exists between helper and seeker of help.

Several times over my career, I have changed the terminology that I use to describe people who enter treatment with me and found myself conflicted even as I wrote this book. Although I was aware of some reservations about using the word "patient," most notably the implication that these individuals are sick, I subordinated these issues to the issue of being able to use my professional power to advocate for the people with whom I was working.

Only recently have I again placed this rationalization under scrutiny. By developing a harm reduction perspective, I have reemphasized my original belief in and respect for the power of the individual to make life choices, even in areas of great potential for harm, such as substance use. I do not necessarily assume that everyone who calls me for consultation is in need of treatment for a serious disorder, or that drug use is inherently good or bad, and I am certainly aware of how much more persons may know about their needs and problems than I do. Yet I resist returning to the word "client." I am also aware of the implications of using a medical model term in a grassroots, consumer-oriented movement such as harm reduction. Still, I prefer the term "patient" to refer to those people who seek my help with drug-related problems.

The only sense that I can make of my language preference is that I actually wear different professional hats in different situations with different people. When I am doing a training session for staff or the general public on harm reduction and the philosophy and approaches that stem from it, I generally refer to people as drug "users." This reflects my belief that it is possible to use drugs without negative consequences. I typically also call drug users "consumers," which underscores my belief in the absolute necessity of building services around the expressed needs of those for whom the services are meant. And when a person comes to me concerned about the problems in his life, whether drug related or rooted in depression or psychosis, I call him a "patient." When I call someone my patient, I feel a different, more profound responsibility in my role as therapist. I am aware that this person has come to me in pain and often with a large amount of fear and shame. She is often suffering from multiple problems that have arisen over many years. At the time she calls me, a crisis has pushed her beyond her usual coping abilities and she is quite vulnerable. At that moment, she is unable to access her own strengths toward helping herself; I promise to offer myself as an anchor and as an active helper, realizing her vulnerability and taking care not to use it to demean her or gain control over her life. Some-

how, for me, the word "client" does not convey this sense of awe-
some responsibility, respect, and intimacy. Nevertheless, I still sometimes use the word "client" rather than "patient." Both terms appear
in this book, and there is no particular pattern to the use of one or
the other.

This book is an explication of a psychotherapy model. It is
organized to draw the reader into the complex issues of drug use in
our society and how our treatment models are dictated by and reflect
societal concerns. Because I view addictions as biopsychosocial
phenomena, a clinical model must include an evaluation of each
component as it affects the person's drug use patterns and history.
Chapter 1 discusses the general principles of harm reduction and
challenges readers to examine their own beliefs about the use of
drugs, the language that we use to talk about people who use drugs,
and the complex history of drug use in the United States. I also offer
epidemiological information to clear up misconceptions about who
uses drugs and to what extent drug abuse is a problem in this
country. I want the reader to understand that there is a significant
relationship between societal attitudes, treatment practices, and
countertransference in psychotherapy.

Chapter 2 introduces the two prevalent models of addiction—
disease and adaptive addiction—and compares the basic tenets of
each. This chapter also uses a case to illustrate the principles of harm
reduction psychotherapy and to discuss some of the general clinical
issues.

In Chapter 3, I introduce a formal assessment process and follow
the case of one particular woman through the entire evaluation to
help the reader see how each element in the Multidisciplinary Assessment Profile (MAP) works in practice.

Chapter 4 describes the process of psychotherapy using harm reduction and then discusses several important psychological dimensions of people with addictive problems. The nature of trust between
therapist and patient is examined, followed by a discussion of three
aspects of psychological life: attachment, affect, and coping skills.
Because I believe addictions are a biopsychosocial phenomenon, I
have included a brief section on neurobiology as it affects addiction
potential.

Chapter 5 is devoted to details of harm reduction psychotherapy with several people. I continue with the case of Joan from Chapter 3 to show how treatment progresses over time. The rest of this chapter is devoted to case studies showing the range of technical possibilities within this model.

Even though I assume that many people with serious drug disorders have significant emotional problems, I specifically address dual diagnosis in Chapter 6, offer some assessment protocols, and again use a case study to show treatment in action.

The final chapter deals with integrating harm reduction into existing practice and settings. While Addiction Treatment Alternatives (ATA), the name of the specific harm reduction psychotherapy model that I developed, was specifically meant as a treatment model, it can be used also for other purposes. I report on two consultation projects, one an organizational development project with an HIV housing provider network, and the other a grand rounds clinical presentation. The book ends by pointing out several significant barriers or difficulties in applying this model, including the difficulties some psychodynamic therapists might have altering standard technique in order to conduct this kind of treatment, as well as the ethical considerations inherent in any new therapeutic practice.

The appendices include a primer of the major drugs of abuse and their physiological effects on the body; an extended history of the use of drugs and alcohol in the United States; and a list of alternative self-help groups, professional treatments, and a self-help reading list.

# Contents

## APPENDICES

PART *I*

---

*OVERVIEW OF*
*HARM REDUCTION*
*PSYCHOTHERAPY*

# CHAPTER ONE

# What Is Harm Reduction?

## INTRODUCTION: FIRST, DO NO HARM

Life teaches. This fact is especially important for those of us who work in the field of psychology. Without the experiences of life in and out of "the chair," our theories and research are poor approximations of the internal workings of a person, and even poorer predictors of behavior. Professional competence may not always accompany professional confidence. A willingness to acknowledge being wrong and to let the client lead the way is a lesson learned late by too many clinicians. Yet it is essential to our learning to "think outside the box." Such creative thinking has led many clinicians to develop new approaches for treating people with complex problems, including drug and alcohol abuse.

The newest innovation in the treatment of drug and alcohol problems is called harm reduction psychotherapy (Tatarsky, 1998). This umbrella term refers to several treatment models based on the international public health movement called harm reduction. Common to all of these treatments is the recognition that problems with drugs and alcohol (like other health and social problems) affect not only individuals, but also families and society. Interventions, then, can target any or all of these areas. The primary principle, however, is to accept the fact that people do engage in high-risk behaviors and to commit to helping these people reduce the harm associated with their behavior. Seat belt campaigns, vaccination programs in the schools, and health screening fairs are all examples of public health, harm reduction interventions. Until recently, needle exchange programs have been the only public health activity specifically targeted to drug users.

Recognizing that traditional approaches to drug and alcohol problems are not very effective, mental health clinicians have been engaged in a search for better treatment strategies for people with these problems (see, e.g., Marlatt, 1996; Marlatt & Tapert, 1993). Several principles guide these efforts: First, the clinician should work closely with the stated goals of the client; second, access to treatment should be "low threshold," that is, having few barriers to entry. (Requiring abstinence prior to treatment, a typical rule of drug treatment programs, is a considerable barrier for many drug abusers.) Harm reduction psychotherapy offers mental health clinicians a way to use traditional psychological principles and techniques as well as emergent strategies in their work with patients who present with multiple problems. It has taken many years of trial and error to develop the particular approach discussed in this book, and many patients received less than effective, respectful treatment during the first years. The admonition "First, do no harm" quickly became a guiding principle for me in the development of this clinical treatment model.

> Maria, age 27, came to a community mental health outpatient clinic asking for therapy to help her deal with family problems. She related a series of disturbing incidents. Her husband of 10 years was working too hard and came home every night and drank himself into a relaxed but useless state. She was less and less able to care for their three children by herself. Her husband became angry when she asked for help with the dishes or with bathing the kids. She was uncomfortable with the increased number of times that she had to call her husband's office and make up excuses for why he would be late or was not coming to work at all some days.

I was the director of the clinic at the time Maria called for an appointment and was responsible for staff training and supervision, as well as direct patient service. Within this setting, I used many different theoretical orientations and clinical styles in order to individualize treatment for a wide variety of patients presenting with a wide variety of problems. Since drug and alcohol treatment services were not offered within the mental health system, however, I knew that all I could offer Maria was information and referral to an alcohol and drug treatment program. Her own difficulties seemed to arise primarily from her husband's alcohol problem. From what I had been taught in school, I concluded she was exhibiting classic behaviors that are often termed "codependent": taking full responsibility for the care of their children and protecting her husband from the consequences of his tardiness and absences from work due to hangovers.

After counseling Maria about the harm done to the family by her husband's alcoholism and her typical codependent responses, I then referred her to a local drug treatment program, where she could receive counseling even if her husband refused. I felt I had done a good job of assessment and referral.

Weeks later, when I spoke with the counselor at Maria's drug treatment center, the counselor confirmed my assessment that the husband had a serious alcohol problem and that Maria exhibited codependent behaviors. The counselor said that he was focusing on Maria's "intractable" codependent behaviors by confronting her in both individual and group sessions. Since I was also trained as a marriage and family counselor, I was a bit concerned that his approach lacked a coherent view of the family dynamics and focused only on the wife's complicity. But I was not the expert in alcoholism treatment; he was. So I did not voice my doubts.

Six months later, Maria called to make an appointment for mental health counseling. I picked up her case and met with her for the first time after having made the referral to the alcohol treatment program. She looked tired but otherwise pretty much as I had seen her previously. She thanked me for having referred her to the alcohol program, saying that it had "saved her life" and helped her see the destructive dynamics in which she had played a part. I asked her what I might be able to help her with now, and she stated that although she had learned to stop her rescuing behaviors, the family was in dire straits. With the encouragement of her alcohol counselor and the group members, she had refused to take on many caretaking roles for her husband. When she stopped calling his job to make excuses for his tardiness, he was fired. Despite advice and confrontations from the counselor and the group about how she should divorce her husband, she found that she just could not leave him. After losing his job, the family of five was now dependent on welfare. The husband's recovery was intermittent and Maria was feeling over-whelmed. Evaluation showed Maria to be anxious and dysphoric with insomnia, hopelessness, difficulty concentrating, and irritability with the children. She expressed both fear and resignation regarding her husband's alcoholism and her continued ability to help him and her children.

I was alarmed and distressed. One question was suddenly fore-most in my mind: *What help did I give her?* Her day-to-day life was more dysfunctional than when I had first seen her, and she was clearly more distressed. I was haunted by the healer's promise to *First, do no harm.*

After several other conversations with the staff at the alcohol treatment program, I became convinced that, even though we viewed her behavior as a sign of pathological denial and codependency that supported her husband's denial, I had done a disservice to this fam-ily. Who was served by my actions? What were the benefits? By re-fusing to think "outside the box," I had failed to take into account the *adaptive* nature of Maria's "codependent" behaviors, which had served to shield the family from poverty by protecting her husband's job. By focusing on her as an individual rather than an important member of a family, I failed to see her lifesaving role and instead con-tributed to the ultimate family breakdown. It was the last time I ever mistook adaptive behavior for codependency. It would not be the last time, however, that I failed to see the adaptive nature of drug use itself. Concern about the probable damage done by alcoholism blinded me to the possible damage done by treatment.

## THE PRINCIPLES OF HARM
## REDUCTION PSYCHOTHERAPY

### First, Do No Harm

This may sound obvious, but often chemical dependency treatment uses interventions that can result in harm to the client or her family (as in Maria's case). It is essential that the treatment do no more harm to the person than the drug use. For example, evicting a person for having drugs on the premises may result in criminal incarceration and/or homelessness that is perhaps much more devastating than drug use. Terminating a patient from treatment because he is using or relapsing places him in danger of further deterioration with no support. Hasty diagnosis and unrealistic treatment planning often result in harm being done by the therapist.

## Drug Addiction is a Biopsychosocial Phenomenon

Research indicates that there is no single cause of addiction, nor even that addictions are primarily biological diseases (Degler, 1991; Miller, 1985; Thombs, 1994). While the pharmacological and biological actions of drugs play an important part in drug problems, other factors are of equal or greater importance in the initiation and maintenance of a drug problem. A person must have several different forces acting on him or her to create the conditions necessary for a serious and persistent drug problem. Emotional traits such as risk taking, psychological variables such as depression, and social realities, including lack of education or advancement, combine with the biological actions of drugs within a person who may also have some genetic sensitivities, and can have many adverse results, including drug abuse and persistent addiction. Addiction may be seen as a central activity (Fingarette, 1988), the final common outcome of many different factors and processes within each individual.

## Drug Use Is Initially Adaptive

Whether used for recreation, escape, or mental enhancement, the initial use of drugs is most often adaptive, that is, beneficial *in some way*. A person uses the drug, perhaps only out of curiosity, to gain an effect that is experienced as positive. Those who continue to "chase the first high," and who develop problems associated with continued drug or alcohol use, are typically people who lack a fuller repertoire of adaptive skills than their peers.

## There Is No Inevitable Progression
## from Use to Dependence

Drug users are an extremely heterogeneous group. One-time curiosity seekers, people who seek regular escape from life stresses, stable working people who use mind-altering substances to relax and en-hance social interaction—all of these types experience a diversity of outcomes (Sobell, Cunningham, Sobell, & Toneatto, 1993). Many young people who use drugs or alcohol, perhaps even excessively, stop or moderate their use as they age and find that being high inter-feres with newly adopted values and plans. Raising a family or work-ing hard at career advancement often take the place of routine drug use in many young adults (Peele, 1991). Treatment for those who present with concerns about continued drug use must respect these differences and tailor treatment styles, intensity, and goals to the par-ticular person.

## The Right to Sensitive Treatment

Boilerplate treatments obviously cannot take into account varying levels of interest in and motivation for treatment. Those clients who are willing or easily persuaded to adopt abstinence as an early goal are usually labeled "motivated." Furthermore, acceptance of atten-dance at 12-Step meetings enlarges our positive view of the client and allows clinicians to relax a bit and direct the treatment in a way that is most comfortable for them. This does not, however, necessarily en-sure success. In fact, *the most common outcome of chemical depend-ency treatment is relapse.* Continued abstinence, even after only 2 years, is the exception (Hester & Miller, 1995; Peele, 1991). Public health interventions such as harm reduction allow a menu of services and do not require adherence to one service in order to be eligible for another. Similarly, people with substance use disorders should be of-fered treatment that is respectful of *their* assessment of their own problems and needs, and clinicians must be willing to work on areas of concern to clients that may or may not correspond to their own.

## Development of a Needs Hierarchy

Central to this attitude of respect is the willingness on the part of the therapist to construct a hierarchy of client needs that reflects and ad-dresses his or her most urgent concerns, longer term goals, and strat-egies toward those goals. Client participation in this goal-setting pro-cess correlates consistently with treatment retention and success (Ojehagen & Berglund, 1989; Sanchez-Craig & Lei, 1986; Sobell,

Sobell, Bogardis, Leo, & Skinner, 1992). One person addicted to alcohol might see his or her biggest problem as a lack of education needed to get a job promotion. Another might see child care problems as the primary source of stress. Even though the alcohol might contribute to or cause the stated problem, from the client's point of view, there are other pressing problems. Therapists ignore these other problems at their own peril and often to the detriment of the therapy. While some therapists refuse to treat a person who engages in dangerous, self-destructive behaviors such as suicide attempts or self-mutilation, most would not refuse treatment to a person who drives too fast or marries an abusive partner. What is the difference except degree of danger? Helping people make connections among their complex attitudes and behaviors, and change is the work of psychotherapy—work that is best done in an interactive rather than dogmatic format. Constructing a needs hierarchy allows patients to assess the many facets in their lives and share with us their values and worries in a way that creates mutual trust and respect.

## Active Drug Users Can and Do Participate in Treatment

Without this belief, borne out in my clinical experience, I could not work with drug users in any creative way. Despite the compulsive, repetitious nature of serious alcohol and drug problems, most people can take steps toward change if they have an active and empathic therapist. Lack of treatment success is often a result of exaggerated expectations of total abstinence from all drugs as the first goal of treatment, as well as the clinician's skepticism about the client really wanting help. Such countertransference positions need to be examined and removed in order to begin treatment that will result in a cooperative working alliance.

## Success Is Related to Self-Efficacy

Just as in other areas of behavior change, success in solving drug-related problems is a function of the client's belief in his or her own power to effect change. Traditional 12-Step approaches that stress the powerlessness of the person over drug use rely on the client's belief in a spiritual being who holds the power to make him or her change. The source of power is located outside of oneself, but power, nonetheless, is seen as essential. Anecdotal evidence and the testimonials of people for whom 12-Step approaches have been successful do not alter the research findings that consistently show that people are more likely to initiate and maintain behavioral changes if they have both a say in the goals and the power to enact them.

## Drug, Set, and Setting: The Client's Unique Relationship with Each Drug Used

Since every drug has its own pharmacology and can be used for different reasons, clients may have very different ways of using and depending upon different drugs. It is common for a person who is abusing alcohol to smoke marijuana occasionally, with no apparent harm. A speed addict may also be physically dependent on Valium but use this second drug only for the muscle spasms that are side effects of speed. Still another person, who may ordinarily drink alcohol in moderation, will when depressed begin a pattern of binge drinking. Research in the area termed a "drug, set, and setting" (Zinberg, 1984) identified the interaction between these three factors in the initiation and maintenance of controlled drug use. *Drug* refers to the actions, or pharmacology of the drug itself, and includes considerations of potency, route of administration, adulterants, and legality. *Set* describes the personality of the person using the drug and includes concepts such as risk taking, mood, motivation (why the person is using right now), expectancy (what the person expects to get from using right now), and emotional problems. Finally, *setting* refers to the context of drug use and includes the location and whether the person is using alone or with others, whether those others are trusted friends or strangers, and, again, the legal status of the drug being used. These three elements interact for each person at each instance of drug use and provide potent information for the patient and clinician.

Therapists who attempt to lump all drug use together, with no regard for these factors, will be unable to decipher the complexities of the person's relationships to different drugs, resulting in an increased chance for misunderstanding and poor treatment outcome.

## Any Reduction in Drug-Related Harm
## Is a Step in the Right Direction

In developing goals and a treatment plan, one should keep in mind that harm reduction psychotherapy, like "regular" psychotherapy, engages the person in a process of incremental change. Evaluating success is often an arbitrary process except in some behavioral interventions. The best guide for monitoring treatment effectiveness is to delineate the specific harms associated with the person's drug use and count any reduction as a success, "a step in the right direction" (Marlatt & Tapert, 1993).

In summary, since addiction is a biopsychosocial phenomenon, in harm reduction psychotherapy, we look for the internal and external factors that initiate and maintain alcohol and drug problems, and create the climate for relapse. By combining research data, client information, and therapist expertise, it is possible to create individualized, effective treatment strategies. Just as we cannot be too frightened by a suicidal client to work effectively with him or her, we have to put aside our fears of the dangers of drug addiction in order to create a treatment that will ultimately free the person from the problem.

## THE MORAL QUESTION:
## IS IT OKAY TO GET HIGH?

Although alcohol and drugs have been used by all cultures for thousands of years, there appears to be a fundamental question about the use of any intoxicant in U.S. society. *Is it okay to get high?*

Patterns of drug use have changed over time and are the product of interacting social, political, religious, and economic forces. Alcohol, usually in the form of beer and other malt beverages, was used by people of many cultures, from ancient civilizations to modern times. In medieval and renaissance England, the daily allotment of beer was one gallon each day for every man, woman, and child (Manchester, 1992). The reasons for this practice most likely include the euphoric effects of alcohol, its pain-killing properties, and the uncertain water quality that was found in ponds and slow-moving streams. Drugs, of course, have an equally long history of use, particularly in religious ceremonies and in shamanic traditions. In addition, people have used stimulants, most notably coca leaves (which contain the drug cocaine) in South America, to increase stamina during heavy work.

It is interesting to note that there has always been a debate about alcohol in the United States. With the exception of certain religious sects, Colonial Americans drank heavily. In general, Fundamentalist Christians deplored drinking, but as America was colonized by more diverse groups, the national consensus appeared to be that alcohol was a regular, normal part of the culture. As socioeconomic and political conditions changed with the Industrial Revolution, so did the apparent consensus. Temperance organizations brought the debate about alcohol use back to the public eye, and people became convinced that alcohol was indeed an evil spirit. This led to the prohibition of beverage alcohol for 13 years. Since then, the national consensus has returned to the belief that alcohol consumption, when moderate, is a normal part of life for most people.

Medicinal tonics, while used by all Americans, were especially prevalent among middle- and upper-middle-class women, who were seen as particularly fragile and in need of medicinal "boosting." These tonics, usually containing alcohol, cocaine, and tincture of opium, were used liberally. Once the reality of physical dependence on these opiate-based tonics became obvious, steps were taken to control their use, and enacted laws resulted in criminalizing people who became addicted or used these drugs without medical supervision. Not only medical practice but also international political forces and the influence of racial prejudice within the United States lay at the heart of drug laws (Musto, 1987).

An individual who uses drugs or alcohol does so within a social context that is defined and limited by the current mores of society. Only occasionally will a radical reorganization of these mores take place. Prohibition banned alcoholic beverages during a time when Americans had become convinced that alcohol was an evil poison. The law was rescinded only 13 years later, and alcohol was returned to a legal place in American social life, despite continued ambivalence toward its use. The 1960s saw dramatic changes in patterns of use and attitudes toward drugs. A large minority saw experimentation with different types of mind-altering drugs as a part of the restructuring of society, not just individual consciousness.

That decade or so of experimentation gave way to stricter controls and to the War on Drugs. Narcotics control has a long history in this country (Musto, 1987), beginning with relationship between the United States and China, and the banning of opium for smoking, continuing to the current interdiction campaigns carried out in Mexico and Peru. Cocaine, and crack cocaine in particular, the demon drugs of the 1980s and 1990s, are seen as being used primarily by racial minorities who then bear the brunt of the drug itself as well as societal legal and moral attacks (Reinarman & Levine, 1997). The intensity of the reactions of those in the mainstream to stories of crack cocaine–using mothers reflects the demonization of crack, black Americans, and women. Harsh penalties for drugs, while they seem morally strong, are in fact politically or racially motivated.

Behind the history, the laws, and the realities of drug use lies a central question that each of us must answer: *Is it okay to get high?* Is it permissible to alter one's consciousness for the purpose of pleasure, religious experience, relief from pain, or escape from reality? If so, for whom is it okay? Under what conditions and with whose permission? What types of mind altering chemicals should be allowed?

At this point, alcohol, nicotine, and caffeine are all legal psychoactive drugs. While a person certainly may like the taste of wine, it would be disingenuous to insist that he or she drinks wine only for the taste and not also for the effect of altering his or her consciousness (or whatever euphemism is used—relax, unwind, etc.). People are quite open about using the stimulant drug caffeine to help them wake up in the morning or renew their cognitive focus in the afternoon. Nicotine, while increasingly recognized as extremely dangerous, is still a legal drug. No one would argue that these legal drugs (perhaps caffeine is an exception) are not capable of causing great harm to the user and his or her family and society. In fact, alcohol and tobacco cause higher rates of morbidity and mortality than do all illegal drugs combined (Frances & Miller, 1998).

In addition to being politically and racially motivated, the differentiation of our reactions to legal versus illegal drugs is related to other components of our culture. For example, legal drugs do not have a counterculture of users and suppliers as does marijuana or heroin. Yet the laws against such drugs have created the counterculture. (Remember the culture of the speakeasy during Prohibition and the rise of organized crime to produce and distribute this illegal drug.) At this point, however, we are used to the dangers of alcohol and hold some belief that we can control those dangers more than we can those of LSD or heroin, for instance. Despite the fact that heroin has few negative physical effects on the body even after long-term use, it continues to be seen as a drug that kills (see Appendix A).

Another difference between legal and illegal drug use is that we have built a benign environment for the consumption of legal drugs; we accept that people enjoy them, we make them readily available in different varieties, and we monitor potency and quality. The shift in public acceptance of nicotine is an example of changing attitudes based on the recognition of the harmful effects of nicotine products. We can easily see the effects on laws, accessibility, and acceptance of use. At the same time that cigars are increasing in popularity, it has become illegal to light up in bars or restaurants in California and many other places across the country. Public opinion has changed the once benign environment of legal nicotine use into a battlefield over public health concerns and individual rights. Smokers are now looked upon with disdain (or pity, if seen as innocent addict–victims of the tobacco industry). The demonization of yet another drug and the isolation of another group of people may well be under way.

This discussion is not offered as an argument for the legalization of any more psychoactive drugs, or for the criminalization of drugs that are now legal. It is intended as an invitation to explore the nature of our attitudes toward drugs in general and our parallel attitudes toward drug users in particular. As clinicians, we are not immune to the biases of our own culture. It is my contention that cultural beliefs, policies, and laws actually form an important basis for what we term "countertransference" in our work with drug users. In psychotherapy, countertransference refers to different aspects of the therapist's reactions to the patient. Initially seen as those reactions based on unresolved pathological elements within the therapist, countertransference is increasingly viewed as a window into the feelings and experiences of our patients (Grayer & Sax, 1986).

This view is interesting. It is certainly useful, and may even be accurate, to read our reactions to patients as indications of their internal life, but we are also feeling the internalized stigma they feel because of societal attitudes toward drug users. Our feelings of disgust or fear, or helplessness, then, may represent more than just the patients' internal associations or our own attitudes. We may be joining patients in a mutual display of society's attitudes toward them. Rather than being in some state of therapeutic neutrality, our patients' feelings, and our own that arise in the treatment setting, most often reflect what we have learned to believe as part of our general cultural indoctrination. Sorting through our own beliefs about the morality of getting high on drugs is imperative if we are to avoid a countertransferential mire of reflected negative judgments and basic misunderstandings of our patients. Such attitude adjustment is the first job of any therapist working with people who use drugs.

Robert, age 37, asked to see a therapist to help him deal with the loss of his wife, who 6 months previously had died of cancer. He was experiencing typical symptoms of grief and felt that he needed some help putting it all into perspective. A history revealed that he had been smoking marijuana three to four times per week since he was 20 years old. His usual pattern was to smoke a few hits from a pipe after coming home from work, eat dinner, and then spend the evening doing whatever he had to do. He reported that since his wife's death, he had been smoking every day, and often in greater quantities than before. He would get stoned and listen to music or just wander around his big house thinking about his wife. He was having trouble keeping up with housework and paying bills, but he continued to work and perform fairly well.

While talking with Robert, I concluded that despite his significant depression, he would probably benefit more from a grief group than from individual therapy. His emotional issues were similar to those of others in his position, and he was not exhibiting any symptoms of pathological grief, such as suicidality or excessive guilt. I was also concerned about his use of marijuana. I stressed to him the importance of quitting the marijuana, but he was resistant to the idea. He perceived that it was not a problem, even though he acknowledged that his use had increased and he was concerned about that. He saw it as a sign of depression.

I agreed with him, but could not say so. I felt constrained by the then-current chemical dependency theory that regular use of any psychoactive drug was indicative of an addictive problem and that depression could not be diagnosed in the presence of active drug use. I strongly suggested to him that he might be in denial about the importance of the marijuana use and that we should continue to talk about it before I could make an assessment and referral to a grief group, since the groups that I had contacted refused to work with anyone who was actively "using."

Robert came to one more session, during which we talked about his wife a little bit, but I kept bringing him back to his increased use of marijuana. Robert canceled the next appointment, saying that he did not feel that the therapy was helping. Once again, I was left with questions: *What help had I given him? What harm had I done?* This was a man in pain because of a traumatic loss. He had sought refuge in his relationship with an old friend, marijuana. My professional point of view at the time would not allow me to view marijuana use in this light. Nor could I allow that perhaps Robert could, in fact, deal with his significant feelings of grief despite the drug use. Seeing drug use as an attachment and a coping strategy was years away for me, both personally and professionally. My view at the time was that for my patients presenting with emotional problems, it was not okay to get high.

## EPIDEMIOLOGY: WHO ARE THESE PEOPLE?

Beliefs about the acceptability, dangers, and morality of drug use often exist in the midst of misinformation and misperceptions about who exactly is doing drugs and how many drug users there really are. The media often give the impression that young people in the suburbs are drinking and using drugs in epidemic numbers. The image of young, urban blacks smoking crack is so prevalent that we tend to overestimate the actual use. These myths and images form part of our belief system about the nature of drug users and thus affect not only public policy, but also our countertransference.

While it is clearly important that our ideas conform more to facts than beliefs, it is very difficult to sort through the various reports on prevalence of alcohol and drug use in the United States. In research, methodological differences, including sample size, diversity of research participants, and whether the study looks at a clinical sample or a cohort from the general population, can confound results and make comparisons of different studies very confusing. Results of studies that are in direct contradiction with others can be used by people with different agendas regarding drug policy and treatment. Although data can be found to support almost any position one might want to take, the larger studies offer the best chance of giving a realistic picture of drug use and drug problems (Kessler, Crum, Warner, & Nelson, 1997). This section describes some of the data on prevalence of both use and substance use disorders taken from large, well-designed studies. Current use and lifetime prevalence of disorders are broken down by gender, race, education, and, sometimes, employment factors. I then present data regarding the typical course of drug use from initiation to dependence and comment on vulnerability factors. Finally, I detail prevalence rates for the major mental disorders as a point of reference.

## Prevalence of Alcohol and Drug Use in the General Population

How many people in this country are using drugs or alcohol on any given day, and what is their typical pattern of use? The 1995 National Household Survey (Substance Abuse and Mental Health Services Administration, 1996) reports on alcohol and drug use by people over the age of 12. In terms of alcohol use, more than 50% of all adult Americans drink (111 million), with 5% showing heavy use and 16% showing binge drinking. These heavy and binge drinkers are much more likely also to use illicit drugs than are other drinkers. Between 18% and 25% of these drinkers will use drugs. More men than women drink alcohol (60% vs. 45%), as do more whites than Hispanics or blacks (56% vs. 45% and 41%, respectively). Illicit drug use follows a different pattern in many areas, educational achievement being the easiest to ascertain. Educational level is related to drug use differently than it is to alcohol. The higher the level of education, the more likely that a person will drink alcohol, but the less likely he or she will use illicit drugs. Whereas half of all the people in this study said that they had tried drugs, only 6% of college graduates currently use drugs, compared to 15% of persons who did not finish high school.

Media headlines notwithstanding, the actual use of illicit drugs in the United States is not increasing in general. The 1995 Household Survey (Substance Abuse and Mental Health Services Administration, 1996) found that almost 13 million people (6%) in the United States were using drugs at the time of the interview, and the vast majority of them were using marijuana (77%). While some of these pot smokers used other drugs as well, more than half used only marijuana. This compares with a high of 25 million drug users in 1979, then a general decline until 1992, when use rose once again, stabilizing for the past 3 years at the current rate. The trend among youth, however, is much different. The rate of drug or alcohol use by young people in the United States has doubled since 1992.

Demographics account for differences in illicit drugs as well as alcohol. Twice as many men as women use drugs, with men preferring stimulants and heroin, and women preferring anxiolytics (such as Valium) and sedatives. There are small but significant differences in racial breakdown, with 8% of African American adults reporting drug use, compared to 6% of whites and 5% of Hispanics. This difference holds true only for adults, however. Adolescents in all three groups have similar rates of use (from 3% to 11%, depending on source of data), suggesting either that a new configuration is occurring or that racially based drug use patterns change as the person ages.

Not surprisingly, level of employment has a strong association with drug use. People who are unemployed are three times more likely to use drugs than those who are employed full time (15% vs. 5%). It is important to note, though, that the vast majority of drug users are actively working (71%), most of them full time. One interpretation of these data is that drug use does not necessarily mean that a person cannot be a productive member of society, but being cut off from productivity is a potent factor in the use of illicit drugs (these data do not tell us whether drug use or unemployment came first).

Age appears to be a limiting factor in the use of drugs and alcohol. One longitudinal study showed no initiation into alcohol or cigarette use after the age of 29, and very little first-time use of any other drugs after that age. In fact, most people stopped using illicit drugs by the age of 29. Daily users of alcohol and also marijuana decreased their use by this age. Only cigarette smokers continued to use and increase daily use with age (Chen & Kandel, 1995).

## Prevalence of Alcohol and Drug Use Disorders

While current usage patterns provide us with a look at the culture in which we live, these data do not address the problems associated with alcohol or drug use. The harm done to individuals, families, and the larger society is most often associated with drug use disorders rather than with casual use (although overdoses on heroin are often associated with new users who have not developed a tolerance). Statistics on drug-related accidents and deaths, while alarming, do not tell us whether the people involved had substance use disorders or fell victim while using at a certain time but had no other substance-related problems. Information on morbidity (illness or accident) and mortality (deaths) must be read with this in mind. The American Psychiatric Association's (1995) practice guidelines for working with people with substance use disorders estimate that 40% of all hospital admissions are directly or indirectly related to alcohol or substance use, and drug use is responsible for up to 25% of all deaths (100,000 deaths per year directly caused by drugs). The majority of these direct deaths are cocaine related and affect black men between the ages of 30 and 39 more often than other groups of people. Intravenous drug use accounts for at least one-third of new HIV cases in the United States, causing illness, and economic and emotional problems for those affected, their families, and society. Medical repercussions of drug use are seen in women and children as well. Up to 15% of pregnant women have used illicit drugs during a pregnancy, and many more have used alcohol during that time.

Given these statistics, how can one view the overall picture of alcohol and drug use problems in this society? The National Comorbidity Study (Anthony, Warner, & Kessler, 1994/1997) reports statistics based on a well-designed study that included 8,000 participants. This study determined the lifetime prevalence of DSM-III-R (American Psychiatric Association, 1994) diagnosed substance use disorders and pointed out several important demographic differences. DSM-III-R definitions require the presence of three out of nine signs and symptoms reflecting the negative consequences experienced by the drug user in order to make the diagnosis. These include continued use despite negative experiences, unsuccessful attempts to quit or cut down, withdrawal symptoms, and so forth. In addition, the problems must have been present for at least 1 month or have recurred several times in one's life. Anyone with such a diagnosis can be viewed as suffering harm and perhaps causing collateral harm as well. Table 1.1 allows easy viewing of information about the prevalence of various substance-related disorders in the general population of the United States. Note that the numbers are rounded and may not add up to 100%.

As in previously cited studies, men are more likely to have a substance use disorder than women. Tobacco dependence is the exception, with rates for females nearing those for men. People ages 25 to 44 make up the largest group with alcohol and illicit drug disorders, whereas older Americans suffer more from tobacco dependence. Contrary to popular images, African Americans are less likely to be drug or alcohol dependent than whites. Hispanics have low levels of tobacco dependence but are similar to whites for all other drugs. The rates of alcohol disorders among Native American peoples are consistently higher than for any other group but vary widely from tribe to tribe. Westermeyer (1996) reports on several studies that found rates of lifetime prevalence anywhere from 25% to 60% for Native Americans and showed serious morbidity and mortality associated with these high rates.

Finally, as in drug use in the general population, employment and education are significantly correlated with substance use disorders. Dependence is most likely to affect unemployed people, those

**TABLE 1.1. Prevalence of Drug Use Disorders**

| Drug type | Lifetime prevalence of disorder |
|---|---|
| Tobacco | 24% (1 in 4) |
| Alcohol | 14% (1 in 7) |
| Other drugs (all) | 7.5% (1 in 13) |
| Cannabis | 4.2% |
| Cocaine | 2.7% |
| Stimulants | 1.7% |
| Anxiolytics/sedatives | 1.2% |
| Heroin | 0.4% |

with lower educational levels, and those making under $20,000 per year.

## Prevalence Comparison of Drug and Psychiatric Disorders

Mental health practitioners often have a skewed perception of the relative incidence of drug use disorders and psychiatric disorders, resulting partly from media emphasis and partly from sampling bias. Most of our patients come to us for emotional problems even if they also have some drug problems. We tend to think of drug problems as occurring on a larger playing field and having greater negative impact on peoples lives than do emotional problems. For instance, we tend to think that addiction to antianxiety drugs such as Valium is very prevalent, and yet it is no more common than is schizophrenia. Similarly, we are led to believe that cocaine abuse is rampant, yet depression is more common. Despite the fact that up to 70% of drug users are employed, we tend to think of these people as unable to work. A look at the incidence of different disorders (see Table 1.2) gives us a perspective on this issue.

These comments do not imply any correlation between the psychiatric disorder and the drug mentioned, only that the incidence is similar for each. Nor is it a comparison of relative harm done by the different problems. In addition, these statistics are not related to the incidence of dual disorders, a topic that will be covered in Chapter 6. Assessing the relative impact of emotional, social, and biological factors is the topic for the Chapter 3.

TABLE 1.2. Comparison of Psychiatric and Drug Use Disorders

| Psychiatric disorder | Prevalence | Comparison drug disorder (abuse or dependence) |
|---|---|---|
| Schizophrenia | 1.2% | Similar to antianxiety agents |
| Bipolar disorder | 1.6% | Similar to stimulants |
| Generalized anxiety disorders | 5.1% | More common than pot |
| Panic disorder | 3.5% } | More common than cocaine, |
| Antisocial personality disorder | 3.5% } | stimulants, sedatives, heroin |
| Simple phobia | 11% | Similar to alcohol |
| Social phobia | 13% | Similar to alcohol |
| Major depression | 17% | More common than any drug problem other than tobacco |

## The Course of Addiction: From Use to Dependence

Even with the previous data, it is still unclear how many people who have used drugs will go on to develop drug disorders. Popular conceptions are that anyone who uses the most addicting drugs (heroin, cocaine, tobacco) is bound to develop dependence, and that almost any drug use is likely to result in significant problems. Many people also believe that the use of marijuana leads to other drug use. Common observation, however, shows that some people seem to be able to use alcohol or other drugs several times with no apparent addictive problem, and others can even use regularly with no apparent harm (Glantz & Pickens, 1992). Alcohol is the best example of this phenomenon among legal drugs, while marijuana fits this profile in the illicit drug category.

Lifetime prevalence data cannot provide information regarding who among all drug users will develop problems. The National Comorbidity Study (Anthony et al., 1994/1997) gathered information that can be used to measure the differences between the numbers of people who use a certain drug and the numbers of those people who eventually become dependent on that drug (see Table 1.3).

These data are surprising enough to be almost unbelievable and certainly contradict popular opinion. Even with drugs known for their addictive potential (heroin and cocaine), fewer than one-fourth of users become dependent. How can we account for this information? First, more familiar research results most often come from treatment samples, people who have *already* developed drug problems. The use of clients to assess the development of a drug disorder is obviously biased given the universal outcome in the sample. Sec-

TABLE 1.3. How Many Drug Users Develop Dependence

| Drug type | Have used drug[a] | Dependence |
|-----------|-------------------|------------|
| Tobacco | 75% | 32% |
| Alcohol | 91% | 15% (21% men, 9% women) |
| All drugs | 51% | 18% |
|    Cannabis | 46% | 9% (1 addict per 10 users) |
|    Cocaine | 16% | 17% (1 addict per 5 users) |
|    Speed | 15% | 11% |
|    Anxiolytics | 13% | 9% |
|    Heroin | 1.5% | 23% (1 addict per 4 users) |

[a]Numbers are rounded.

ond, there must be certain presently unknown factors that increase or decrease the risk of using a drug and perhaps different factors that are related to eventual dependence. In other words, there may be particular vulnerabilities in a person that we can cite as predictors of drug dependence. Many researchers are studying this problem, as it appears to be the best way to develop prevention and early intervention strategies.

## Vulnerability to Drug Problems

In terms of identified risk factors, gender is an obvious one. Men are more likely to use and become dependent on alcohol and cannabis, whereas women are more likely to use and become dependent on anxiolytics and sedatives. As mentioned earlier, use of tobacco among women has increased dramatically over the past 10 years, men and women being almost equal in prevalence of use and addiction. Factors of underemployment and lack of educational achievement have also been mentioned. Early onset of drug use predicts greater dependence. Young adults, ages 15–24, who use cocaine become dependent at a rate of 25%, whereas of those first-time users ages 25–44, only 15% become dependent (Anthony et al., 1994/ 1997).

Perhaps developmental factors play an important role as well. One project involved research using drug histories from 1,200 young adults in the New York State Follow-Up Cohort (Kandel & Davies, 1992). Using marijuana as the target drug, researchers obtained risk factors for the progression from initial use to near-daily use (defined as marijuana use 20 out of every 30 days). These risk factors include having a family member who had been treated for any emotional problems, poor grades in school, early onset of use (age 13 rather than 17), and having a father who was a heavy drinker while the child was in high school. In addition, the study found that episodes of near-daily marijuana use typically first occur between the ages of 19 and 20 and last over 3 years. Another interesting finding is that over time, these near-daily users tend to reduce both the frequency and the quantity of marijuana used, supporting other research that indicates that *the highest use of most drugs, not just marijuana, occurs early in life, with spontaneous remission being the rule rather than the exception.* Tobacco is the only drug for which this is not the case.

Factors that affect vulnerability to continued drug problems are likely to be different for different racial groups. Research on drug use by African Americans yields contradictory information. While the previously cited Household survey (Substance Abuse and Mental Health Services Administration, 1996) indicates lower drug use rates for blacks than for whites, many other investigators have found higher rates. Brunswick, Messeri, and Titus (1982) conducted a large study that focused primarily on identifying factors that could predict adult drug use in a group of African American adolescent drug users. They tested a "developmental ecological model" (p. 420) by combining concepts from social learning theory and social control theory to create research dimensions such as social bond and social structure. Their results show that social class, peer pressure, age of initiation into drug use, and occupational status combine in complex ways to create an individual who may initiate drug use while young and either stop it or progress to serious use in adult life. In addition, gender plays an important role in the relative influence of these different factors.

What other influences, separately or together, combine to increase vulnerability to the transition from use to drug addiction? The authors of the National Comorbidity Study summed up their data by stating that "considered all together, the array of theoretically plausible determinants of the transition from drug use to drug dependence runs the span from the microscopic (e.g., the dopamine receptor) through the macroscopic (social norms for or against drug use; international drug-control policies)" (Anthony et al., 1997, p. 32). Clearly, drug use and drug dependence are complex biopsychosocial behaviors that interact in predictable and unpredictable ways. More of these factors are discussed in Chapter 4.

## THE NATURE OF SUCCESS REDEFINED

Harm reduction psychotherapy allows clinicians to perceive and define success in radically different ways. My patients have become significantly better. Not all improved greatly regarding the use of substances, but many became abstinent after long periods of time during which they were attempting to learn moderation. Others had stable housing and finances but were actively using and expressed little desire to quit. An encouraging number of others eliminated the problems that brought them into treatment by modifying their drug or alcohol use. I realize that for them and for me, the definition of "success" had changed. I now define "success" as any movement in the direction of positive change, any reduction in drug-related harm.

People have the right to make their own decisions in life. I first developed this conviction while working with psychiatric patients. I learned that what works best is offering what I can in the moment and standing by while they live their lives outside the therapy hour. I have witnessed the continuum of healthy to risky lifestyle choices in all of my clients, and respecting my clients' decisions works equally well when these people have substance use disorders. The fact that they may make treatment choices and life choices that conflict with my professional or personal beliefs does not relieve me of my responsibility to offer them what help I can.

Tina was a 24-year-old woman hospitalized with a diagnosis of schizoaffective disorder. She was taking Navane, an antipsychotic drug, and had a long history of emergency room contacts that once before had resulted in inpatient treatment. She was currently homeless. She had never followed up with outpatient referrals, so I decided to see her first while she was still in the hospital, hoping that this connection would facilitate her transition into outpatient care. This strategy worked and she did present at the outpatient clinic, where a comprehensive history revealed amphetamine and marijuana use over a long period of time. She did not use daily, she said, but only when someone gave her drugs or she had money.

Concerned that some of her symptoms were caused by her drug use, I consulted with a local drug treatment program. I was told that speed use can also cause psychotic symptoms, and that there was no point in trying to treat her until she was clean of all drugs, including the Navane, for at least 30 days. While I was reluctant to discontinue the Navane, the other advice seemed reasonable to me and I expected no objection from the patient. Terminating treatment temporarily might be difficult because we had seen each other four or five times by then, and Tina seemed to feel connected to me. But I was not prepared for the anger she hurled at me when I told her that I could not see her in the clinic until she had completed a 30-day drug program.

Because she was still a little psychotic, I assessed her paranoid thought that the "system is working to send me away" as just psychotic process. Tina left the session early and did not return, nor did she present at the drug program. She was admitted to the hospital 3 weeks later after a serious suicide attempt prompted by hallucinatory voices.

Once again, I asked myself what good I had done. More importantly, *what harm had I done?* A more *successful* outcome for Tina might have occurred if I had kept her *in* psychotherapy as a way of addressing her drug problems. Obviously, a more *successful* outcome would have been to prevent a suicide attempt by offering continued contact and support.

The concepts and applications outlined in this chapter offer the clinician a snapshot of the complexities involved in designing treatment for people with substance use disorders. In choosing a harm reduction approach, one can then "test" any given intervention against the principles involved. Most clinicians fall on different ends of the harm reduction spectrum. It is not really possible to be for or against harm reduction. Harm reduction is what we do all the time. The only decision is how many of the principles one embraces and how far one is willing to allow the client to dictate the course and goals of treatment. This flexibility allows many more clinicians to enter the substance use field and contribute ideas and criticisms that enrich this new model of treatment.

# CHAPTER Two

# The Development of Harm Reduction Psychotherapy

*T*he three cases in the previous chapter exemplify the professional struggle that gave rise to this book. In each case, my therapeutic interventions caused more harm to my patients than did the drugs they were using. This chapter offers the reader a comparison of the different viewpoints on addiction and a new way of looking at these problems.

## THE BASIC MODELS AND VIEWPOINTS ON ADDICTION

The two current major theoretical orientations regarding the nature of addiction are the *disease model* and several other models, collectively called *adaptive models* (Alexander, 1987). They differ primarily in the weight given to biological versus psychological factors that initiate and maintain alcohol and drug abuse. Alexander points out that the disease model views the individual as engaging in mechanical, determined behavior, whereas adaptive models stress the purposeful nature of the activity. Therefore, the models also differ significantly regarding treatment philosophy, strategies, and prognosis.

## The Disease Model

Even though the term "disease" was used in reference to alcoholism as early as the 19th century, it was only after the end of Prohibition that a formal disease model replaced the moral model of addiction, which viewed alcoholics as sinful and weak (see Appendix C). This newer model holds that addictions are biological diseases that have no cure, that this disease is characterized by denial, loss of control, and inevitable progression toward death. Recovery is a lifelong process of containment rather than a successful cure. Only certain people have the disease (this has been taken to mean that heavy drinking is not the *cause* of alcoholism; rather, it is the most obvious *symptom* of alcoholism).

The disease model is best represented by Alcoholics Anonymous (AA) and 12-Step programs. It is the dominant philosophy for addiction recovery in the United States but has less following in other countries. AA is a direct result of the temperance movement, specifically the efforts and ideals of the Oxford Group, a Christian fundamentalist businessman's group. Two Oxford group members, Bill Wilson and Bob Smith, MD, founded AA in 1935, just 2 years after the repeal of Prohibition (Bufe, 1991). AA adopted the disease concept and developed the tenets we know today, which combine a biological, quasi-scientific explanation with evangelical Protestant values as the treatment of choice.

### Basic Tenets

The Nature of Addiction

- Addiction is a biological disease that affects only certain people.
- People with addictions are psychologically different from others.
- Denial maintains the disease.
- Loss of control is a symptom of the disease.
- The disease inevitably progresses to death if unchecked.
- Social or psychological issues are largely irrelevant. Problems in living are caused by the disease.
- The disease is transferable from one substance to another (nonspecificity of the disease).

Treatment Implications

- Lifelong abstinence from all psychoactive drugs is the only acceptable treatment.
- Confrontation of denial is essential.
- User must accept being powerless and surrender to a higher power.
- Recovering addicts are the best people to help other addicts.
- No special consideration is given regarding race, gender, ethnicity, and so on. Addiction is assumed to be the same for everyone (an equal-opportunity disease).
- Since there is no cure, a lifelong recovery process is essential to prevent relapse.

As currently practiced, the disease model has changed little since AA originated except that the model has been extended to cover drugs as well as alcohol and, more recently, "process addictions" as well (gambling, overeating, sexual compulsion). Workers in the field are often in recovery themselves. The model assumes that ex-addicts are best able to help other addicts because they have experienced both addiction *and* recovery. However, this subjectivity leads to a stance that is often anti-intellectual and results in clinicians who are often unaware of recent empirical findings about both the nature of addiction and newer treatments that might be useful (Thombs, 1994).

## Adaptive Models

Adaptive model approaches include a collection of separate psychological models that are often used in conjunction with each other.

Alexander (1987) offers an in-depth analysis of the two viewpoints on addiction, the disease model and adaptive models. He describes adaptive model approaches as those that place primary etiological significance on early childhood developmental problems that lead to specific adaptive failures in the young adult or the adolescent. Drug or alcohol abuse is seen as an active, originally adaptive, search for compensatory mechanisms: A girl learns that her shyness can be alleviated by drinking a beer before she goes out; a boy does not feel the pain of a broken relationship if he uses heroin. These compensatory actions of the drug are potent reinforcers. The use of drugs or alcohol stabilizes the person under certain conditions, allowing some measure of normal functioning. Many people remain at this level of use throughout their lifetimes.

For others, though, increases in stress and drug use over time cause the characteristic symptoms that we see in addiction. The person experiences a reemergence of the same difficulties that led to the search for compensatory activities in the first place. Financial, social, and occupational functioning deteriorate as the drug abuse develops *functional autonomy* (a term used to describe how drug abuse eventually becomes unmoored from its origins in emotional underpinnings and takes on a life of its own). The specific pharmacology of the drug also contributes to the types of problems and usually the rate and severity of the eventual addiction. For example, marijuana users generally take a long time to develop negative effects. Crack cocaine, however, can create serious problems immediately, as can phencyclidine (PCP). Alcohol, being legal, may cause serious psychosocial dysfunction but will not result in conflict with the justice system. Heroin use, on the other hand, can result in significant legal problems.

Adaptive models include a range of psychodynamic, cognitive, and behavioral treatments, each based on fundamental beliefs about the nature of human psychopathology, health, and the role of psychotherapy in treatment. These various models are extremely different from each other. Many cognitive and behavioral approaches were developed specifically for work with addictions and have been used in chemical dependency treatment programs for some time. The difference between the disease model and adaptive models is therefore a somewhat blurred but nonetheless important distinction.

### Basic Tenets

The Nature of Addiction

- There may or may not be a genetic component to addictions.
- Drug use often temporarily solves life's problems.
- People develop severe drug problems because they need compensatory adaptations (e.g., they are shy, fatigued, depressed, traumatized).

- Drug users can be understood by the same psychological principles as other people (you do not have to be one to treat one).
- Prolonged drug use can lead to a return of original problems *plus* severe new problems.
- While socioeconomic class, race, and ethnicity are given some practical consideration, overall theory assumes white, male "norms."

Treatment Implications

- Exploration of possible causes in a person's background is important.
- The use of theoretical models developed for other disorders is possible.
- The focus is on affect, thought, and behavior, not drug actions.
- One may or may not use disease model practices.

Despite being different from the disease model, many adaptive models continue to view addictions as diseases. These approaches suffer from the same problems that I encountered in trying to develop an alternative to traditional models: They either ignore the specific drug effects or relegate internal dynamics to the background. No special theory has yet been developed to overcome this conflict. Most recently, psychotherapists from around the United States have been working toward the development of a new paradigm that will shift the focus of drug treatment to the *person* who is using drugs and the community in which he or she lives. The term "harm reduction psychotherapy" (Tatarsky, 1998) has been suggested for this developing model, which has its origins in public health principles, including harm reduction. I describe the most important concepts of public health and then harm reduction, since both form the basis for the development of my treatment approach, Addiction Treatment Alternatives (ATA).

## Public Health Concepts as Foundation and Bridge

Public health models attempt to do the greatest good for the greatest number of people. They are population based rather than focused only on the individual. This approach holds that health exists on a continuum, as do the dangers of ill health. Because one person's problem is the community's problem as well, all efforts are directed at reducing the harm to the community of health problems. The measure of success is the reduction of disease in various areas, not the eradication of disease in all people.

How one views a problem directly affects its solutions. Public health models locate the problem of drug abuse in a biopsychosocial environment, unlike the disease model and some adaptive models, which see the drug abuse as residing only within the individual. This viewpoint then affects how we conceptualize the pathology of drug use and dictates the treatment needed. If addictive disorders reside within individuals, then only individual treatment techniques are necessary. If, however, drug abuse is a complex psychosocial phenomenon, then interventions within the community, as well as for the individual, are necessary to resolve the harm that can be done by excessive drug use.

Public health policy rests on several principles that serve as a theoretical guide and practical assessment strategy of the usefulness of interventions. Of primary importance is needs assessment, a survey of the actual people within a given community, to find out people's perceptions of what services they need and the priorities they would assign to the different possibilities. Their self-identified needs are then combined with professionals' knowledge of health-related problems in this population, and services are developed and implemented, again with continuing input from the consumers, the people in the community who need the services. Once the service is in place, the strategy expands to include techniques to bring people to the service.

The fundamental principle of public health is *low threshold* access (Marlatt & Tapert, 1993). Services are offered with the least amount of requirements or restrictions, so that as many people as possible can take advantage of and benefit from them. Such a philosophy attempts to include many people in treatment in order to reduce harm not only to the individual but also to his or her family and community. The patient has few "hoops" to jump through, often not having to agree to come at a certain time or being asked for identification. Patients are not denied one service because they refused another that was linked to it (e.g., mothers who use drugs can still bring their babies in for vaccinations, and the active alcoholic can be treated for an abscessed tooth). Another common practice in public health services is to provide information as well as services. Booklets and public lectures, for example, offer information so that people can decide what is best for themselves as a result of knowledge.

The HIV epidemic and the resulting challenges by health consumers propelled the public health clinics to provide not only medical care to this group, but also to offer education regarding safe sex practices, to give out free condoms, and to teach people how to clean their "works," the injection equipment used by intravenous drug users. The goal was to reduce the harm caused by these activities, specifically to reduce the spread of HIV. The success of these efforts is well documented.

## Harm Reduction

Harm reduction was first developed in Europe, most notably in the Netherlands, in direct response to the HIV epidemic, which was spread there primarily by intravenous drug users who shared their needles (Springer, 1991). Harm reduction offers both a set of principles and a pragmatic strategy for intervention that directly challenges the usual ideology of addiction treatments. Based on the public health principles discussed earlier, harm reduction focuses its efforts on identifying and reducing drug-related harm, and allows that while abstinence may sometimes be the most certain strategy to protect a person, any move to reduce harm is a step in the right direction and worthy of assistance (Marlatt, 1998a).

Harm reduction addresses the needs of the client, called the user, according to a needs assessment created with the user from the first point of contact. Offered services reflect the needs identified by the drug user—needle exchange, smoking cessation programs, methadone maintenance, family planning, psychotherapy, and so forth. These services, while often controversial, are in the public view. But many harm reduction outreach workers and professional clinicians are often afraid to admit that they practice other clinical interventions, such as controlled drinking strategies, instruction in the moderate of use of amphetamines, training users to switch from injectable drugs to oral use, teaching vein care for intravenous drug users, and other undocumented and unsupported clinical activities.

Harm reduction methods represent a paradigm shift and allow the development of a model that addresses drug users' other needs as well as their drug problems. Educational, parenting, vocational, and basic medical services are, in this view, essential parts of a healthy lifestyle. Unlike some drug rehabilitation programs that offer these services, harm reduction does not require abstinence from drugs in order for patients to take part in these activities. Such a low threshold approach invites the drug user to develop health promotion strategies that may include drug management or abstinence.

Finally, harm reduction psychotherapy bears a close resemblance to the research on relapse prevention, particularly on the concept of self-efficacy, or self-confidence, as an essential tool to initiate and maintain change. Increasing one's sense of personal power leads to more stable behavior changes than approaches that question the abilities of the drug user, as do disease and adaptive models.

### Basic Tenets

The Nature of Addiction

- There is a continuum of drug use from nonproblematic to extremely problematic, and a continuum of harms as well.
- Harm reduction psychotherapy does not enter into the debate of whether drug use is pathological.

Treatment Implications

- Harm reduction psychotherapy accepts the person "where he is."
- The focus is on reducing the harm caused by drug use, not on use per se.
- This approach allows the client to select goals that range from abstinence to safer use of drugs.
- The treatment is based on the rights of individuals to make choices (and their rights to sensitive, appropriate assistance with drug-related problems).
- Cultural, racial, and ethnic differences are incorporated.
- Harm reduction methods are open to professional advice and interventions.
- The methods are based on research in self-efficacy and change.

- Interventions engage users in developing strategies specific to their situation.
- Harm reduction methods acknowledge that the user may have other, more pressing problems than drug use.

These concepts and strategies are currently being used to develop what is being called "harm reduction psychotherapy" for the treatment of drug and alcohol disorders.

The previous section condensed the basic tenets of each approach in ways that allow comparisons of beliefs and the very real differences in interventions that develop out of each belief system. While the disease model offers a coherent, easily applied treatment approach, its lack of individuality and flexibility reduces its appeal and appropriateness for a variety of people seeking help with a drug or alcohol problem. Additionally, it has a low efficacy (approximately a 35% success rate) and so is not a potent intervention in terms of populations despite the fact that it may be decidedly useful for a particular individual. On the other hand, adaptive model adherents are often uninformed about drug effects and tend to view all drug use as merely a symptom of some (more essential) defect or process. Harm reduction therapists offer an attitude of respect and practical strategies for drug users and understand the complex interactions among a person, the environment, and drug use; however, the adaptive model cannot by itself offer an interconnecting theory that will support therapeutic interventions. Harm reduction psychotherapy models offer such a coherent, multidimensional and multidisciplinary approach to the person with a drug or alcohol problem.

## Harm Reduction Psychotherapy

### Basic Tenets

The particular harm reduction approach that I have developed combines the principles of harm reduction with psychodynamic and cognitive models of psychotherapy. The result is a holistic treatment model, based on both empirical and clinical experience, that is pragmatic, flexible, effective, and allows clinicians to treat addicts as people with problems, not as problem people. A reciprocal exchange of practical techniques and conceptual principles enhances the usefulness of this model. My patients open my eyes to experiences that I could not have imagined and suggest solutions that I would not have thought them capable of conceiving. This trust in and respect for the patient is the fundamental principle of any harm reduction approach.

## The Nature of Addiction

- Addictive behaviors are a combination of biopsychosocial forces:
    The relationship between user and the drug of choice
    Self-medication of emotional distress
    Biological vulnerability
    The changes in use over the lifespan
- Drugs are used by many people for many different reasons, and with many different outcomes.
- Addiction is not a disease.
- There is a circular continuum of use—not an inexorable progression—including nonuse, moderate use, or persistent addiction.
- Many people "recover" with little or no help.
- Not all illicit drug use is abuse.
- There are special influences of race, gender, and culture on the development and maintenance of addictions.
- Most people know when they have a drug problem. Shame and public judgments lead to lying and denial.
- Ambivalence about giving up the *benefits* of drug use leads to resistance to change.
- People with problems can participate meaningfully in treatment.
- Drug users can be understood using the same psychological principles as those applied to other people.
- Change occurs as a series of steps, or stages.

## Treatment Implications

- Harm reduction psychotherapy involves a biological and a psychodynamic understanding of the etiology of addiction, a cognitive-behavioral and pharmacological–biological understanding of its maintenance, and an understanding of the functional autonomy of persistent addiction.

- Assessment strategies must include biopsychosocial dimensions.
- Because motivation is a result of the interaction between client and therapist, the development of therapeutic rapport is the foundation of treatment.
- Users can and should participate with the therapist in all phases of treatment, including the mutual development of a needs hierarchy, goals, strategies, and outcome measures.
- The *harm done,* not the drug use itself, is the focus.
- Drug users have needs other than drug treatment; the treatment should focus on these.
- Confrontation is to be avoided.
- Special techniques reduce resistance and increase motivation.
- *Any reduction in drug-related harm is a success* (a change in the right direction).

## DISCUSSION OF THE PRINCIPLES OF HARM REDUCTION PSYCHOTHERAPY

A postcard from a local card shop shows three hypodermic syringes overlaid with the words "100,000 heroin addicts can't be wrong." For many who came of age in the 1960s, it is obvious that drugs are used by many people for many different reasons, and with many different outcomes. The stoned-out hippie who is now a stock broker is a stereotype of the transformation that occurred in the 1980s in our country. The shirt-and-tie engineering student who went through the 1970s mesmerized only by a slide rule, became addicted to cocaine in the 1980s, quit using in the 1990s, and now runs a successful business. And of course, there is the person who started smoking pot and is now on the streets, a junkie with HIV disease.

What differentiates these people? How is it that the use of drugs can be so variable with regard to both personality types and outcome? Everything I had originally been taught indicated that what appear to be different addictions are in fact one unitary disease, pretty much the same for everyone. The individual variability was purported to be merely a "cunning subterfuge" that hides the true nature of addiction, a progressive disease that will prove fatal unless the person abstains from all psychoactive drugs for the rest of his or her life.

The belief that not all drug users will suffer severe consequences led to a companion principle: There is a continuum of drug use that flows from nonuse (abstinence) to use, abuse, addiction, and what Stanton Peele (1991) calls *persistent addiction*. As is the case with other behaviors, the continuum of drug use is not an inevitable progression. Rather, it is a fluid dynamic in which individuals may move in and out of various levels of drug use. For the most part, individuals' positions on the continuum at one point in time do not imply that they will remain there, nor that they will progress to a more harmful point on the continuum. Many people, up to 35% by some accounts, recover with no help from others. Indeed, few people begin using drugs and most people stop by the age of 29. This spontaneous recovery is referred to by Peele (1994) as a process of *maturing out*. Some people grow up and recognize that there are competing values, plans, or responsibilities that discourage their continued use. Others develop problems associated with their drug or alcohol use and decide to make some changes themselves, either using in moderation or quitting. The important lesson is that *most* people make changes toward reducing drug-related harm rather than following a deteriorating course.

Few people know that drugs can be used by many people without progressive deterioration. How is it that this information, important in the development of drug policy and treatment, has not reached the mainstream? After much study of the history of attitudes and laws regarding alcohol and drugs in the United States, it is apparent to me that American attitudes (and policies) are based on misinformation and biases that, while originating in social realities, have become religious, legal, or political in nature, rather than empirical or experiential. The fact is, not all use of illicit drugs can be construed as abuse.

In fact, people who use drugs are often indistinguishable from people who have other kinds of problems. Contrary to the public perception (shared by many professionals) that drug users are high-profile criminals, social pariahs, and misfits, epidemiological data indicates that aside from the illegality of the drugs themselves, many users live within the rules of society and pose no special burden on social or health resources. Those drug users who do require services appear similar to other consumers of public resources such as health care, housing, education, and rehabilitation. Many are no more difficult to deal with than the ordinary citizen, who occasionally misses appointments or forgets to follow the doctor's recommendations. However, the public health system continues to struggle with the problem of attending to the needs of a drug-using population in the current climate of zero-tolerance and the War on Drugs. This negative climate has created a mutual mistrust when drug users try to access services.

The mental health care system has had a particularly difficult time in the adjustment to working with patients with both mental health and substance use problems. It is in this arena that substance-using patients present additional dilemmas. Clinicians are often unaware of the different characteristics and special needs of a drug-using population, including mistrust, baffling symptom complexes, and medical problems secondary to the drug use. Professionals in mental health have shunted drug users into a category of "intractable" patients who are demanding, manipulative, and frustrating. The effort has been to identify and eliminate these patients from treatment rather than to include them and design programs for their special needs. After years of struggling with these attitudes, I realized that quality treatment must be based on the principle that drug users are people with problems, not problem people. The following case illustrates many of the stated principles of harm reduction psychotherapy.

## CASE ILLUSTRATION

Joan, a 27-year-old lesbian, was referred to me by a colleague who did not want to treat her because she was addicted to prescribed pain killers. Joan was not, however, seeking treatment for her drug use, but for relationship problems. On intake, Joan freely admitted to taking six to eight Vicodin each day for the past 6 years. These pills were prescribed by her orthopedic surgeon for hip pain that had resulted in surgery 3 years earlier. Despite the improvement in her hip pain, she continued to use the Vicodin, often taking more than was prescribed and then asking for more from the physician, who complied with her requests. Joan's main concern was that she could not maintain a stable intimate relationship. Her history included abandonment by family, subsequent sexual abuse in an orphanage, and a heroic struggle to put herself through both college and graduate school. She worked hard in a professional job and had been at the same location for 4 years. Joan's narcotic use was not a concern for her, but she had been terminated by two other therapists because she was an "active drug addict." She was confused and somewhat hurt by these rejections.

She reported a series of intense, chaotic attachments to women who quickly tired of her demands for reassurance and constant contact. She became obsessively jealous and at times verbally assaultive if her efforts to control her girlfriend failed.

After two or three sessions in which Joan focused on her relationship concerns, she offered the information that she thought she maybe "drank too much sometimes," often up to a pint of bourbon at a time. She also said that she used cocaine, but mostly for recreation. I asked her, "Mostly?" My question was not addressed until a few sessions later. Joan commented that once this information came out in her previous therapies, the therapists "freaked" about drug addiction and could not talk about anything else.

I had some appreciation of these therapists' dilemma as I found myself silently screaming, "Now what do I do?" My first impulse was to focus on Joan's considerable drug use and her unwillingness to label it as a primary problem. I realized, however, that by doing so, I would merely repeat her previous experiences with therapy (and possibly an important reenactment of her early life). I chose to "do no harm" as a good initial strategy.

Joan exhibited clear signs of borderline personality disorder. Her lifestyle of chaotic relationships, impulse-ridden behavior, affective lability, and externalization of her problems offered a classic presentation of this disorder. Many of her disruptive behaviors occurred after drinking alcohol, but her use of the narcotic Vicodin did not appear at first evaluation to contribute either to her psychological or behavioral problems, since narcotics, in general, do not contribute to either disinhibition nor moodiness. Cocaine, on the other hand, with its intense stimulating effects, could easily cause some of the symptoms Joan was exhibiting. Listening to her describe the emotional events that often preceded her use of these drugs, it became clear that substance use often formed a protective emotional shield around this vulnerable woman. Clearly, though, at times, it also disrupted her fragile equilibrium.

This paradox of adaptive use of drugs co-occurring with significant harm is the basis of a harm reduction perspective. Harm is *one* result of using drugs, but not the *only* possible outcome. Refusal of traditional drug treatment models to allow for this paradox has resulted in a lack of understanding of the real complexities of drug use, and in the development of an negative attitude about the drug user, who often does not see any damage done by her drug use because she is so busy protecting its benefits. Therapists then employ the concept of denial (denial of a problem, denial of having a disease) to simplify what is a complex psychological process that includes both the patient's accurate insight into her drug use *and* a lack of awareness that certain clinical symptoms may be associated with that same use. This ambivalence about drug use is a healthy and honest response for most clients. Refusing to simplify ambivalence by confronting only one side of it ensures that the therapist and client will not be polarized.

In my work with Joan, it was difficult to shift the focus of the therapy to include any meaningful discussion of her drug use. Her current relationship was the source of her worry. She knew that if she could not gain some control over her jealousy, this woman would leave her as others had. From her perspective, drug treatment was not at the top of her *needs hierarchy*. This apparent lack of motivation to address critical issues of addiction was, in fact, a clear statement of motivation to begin work on her core problems—as she saw them. Traditional requirements for the client to address issues as the therapist sees them had already resulted in several treatment failures for this woman. By allowing her to take the lead in her own psychotherapy, she made me realize that drug users *can and do participate meaningfully in their treatment*.

After much soul searching, I decided to work with Joan on her relationship difficulties while paying close attention to any connection between her drug use and the patterns in these relationships. I let Joan know that I was concerned about the possible effects of the drugs on her relationships and she responded with surprise. She had not considered her drug use much of a problem at all and did not see it as interacting with her relationships. I suggested that she begin to pay attention to anything that struck her as connected to these two aspects of her life. In this case, the patient was motivated to work on relationship issues but not to explore her drug use. Pairing the two, however, opened up the possibility of "indirectly" (as I thought about it at the time) working on her drug use. After several months of therapy, Joan began to notice that her worst fights occurred after she had been drinking but not while using other drugs. Together, we developed a plan for her to refrain from drinking on the evenings when she saw her girlfriend. This strategy worked, and Joan began to exercise some control over her alcohol and drug use.

## DISCUSSION OF THE MODEL

This abbreviated description of a prolonged psychotherapy highlights the critical differences between traditional drug and alcohol treatment models and a psychotherapeutic model based on harm reduction principles. By listening to the client and interpreting what one hears through this new filter, it is possible to design truly individualized treatment that increases motivation for change and challenges the client to become a full participant. My experience has shown that when clients are offered this type of therapy, resistances often seen in traditional settings are rendered less potent and can be used constructively as indicators of normal ambivalence in persons who are about to make life-altering changes.

Many clinical experiences, similar to the one with Joan, eventually led me to another cornerstone of harm reduction psychotherapy and yet another disagreement with traditional chemical dependency lore. People can and do make changes in their lives while still using drugs or alcohol, and they do participate in treatment if they are allowed to lead the way.

Terms such as "denial" and "lack of motivation" have been used routinely by people who treat drug users. I believe that these concepts are both inaccurate and often destructive to the therapeutic relationship, especially when used in a pejorative rather than descriptive manner, as if drug users are "deniers" and "treatment lazy." In fact, denial in the clinical setting is actually an indicator of ambivalence rather than a refusal to admit to a problem. As will be discussed in more detail in Chapter 3, ambivalence is a normal, healthy state in which the person tries to weigh the pros and cons of his or her drug use. This process is essential to the development of a solid therapeutic alliance and a working treatment plan.

Most drug users are not in denial. They know they use drugs and, when problems develop, they are aware of those problems. The difficulty for them is to admit it to someone else, particularly someone who is already criticizing them for their behavior. Most of us share this tendency to hide certain negative traits while under public scrutiny. This is not peculiar to drug users. We all hide, minimize, distort, or outright lie about our worst habits or characteristics at times. Creating a therapeutic relationship in which client and clinician engage mutually in an investigative process minimizes this universal human tendency.

A companion concept frequently addressed in chemical dependency programs is the client's lack of motivation, implying that motivation is a stable trait that resides solidly within the individual. Yet Miller and Rollnick (1991) argue persuasively that motivation exists within an interpersonal matrix, and thus is fluid and exquisitely sensitive to interactions between two people. This optimistic viewpoint gives the clinician both power and responsibility to increase motivation for treatment, while removing from the user the stigma of being an uncooperative client. Both parties in the interaction contribute toward positive or negative motivational stances. No longer should we wait until a person "bottoms out" or gets motivated to begin treatment. Increasing motivation for change *is* the work—it does not necessarily occur prior to treatment.

In the past 5 years, published research has periodically reported that the "cause" of alcoholism has been found. The results of genetic, metabolic, and identical twin studies announced with certainty that alcoholism is a biological disease. The only question was which of the many factors were responsible. Upon examination, the research was not impressive. Methodological flaws, the use of only male subjects, samples taken from inpatient programs rather than mixed modalities, or the minimal correlations found in many studies weakened the findings. Several people came forward as critical reviewers of this research (Peele, 1991; Thombs, 1994) and many others joined the discussion about the underlying assumptions of the disease model and the problems inherent in it (Alexander, 1987).

The clinical model in this book emerged as a harm reduction treatment based on the belief that addictions are a complex combination of biopsychosocial forces. There is a relationship between the user and the drug of choice, in which the drug takes on many elements of a primary attachment figure. The user may idolize the drug, only to feel hateful toward it during a hangover or withdrawal. Promises never to do the drug again are reminiscent of a person swearing never to go out with a former lover who treated her badly. Alternately, she may use the drug when she needs reliable relief from stress or boredom. All of these relationship patterns can occur with other people or with drugs. A careful psychosocial history very often reveals clear emotional or social problems for which the person once actively sought solutions, then discovered drugs in her active search for compensatory mechanisms. It is important for the clinician to realize that the drugs worked at least a little, and at least for a while. This is one of those ideas that, once articulated, seems obvious and based in common sense. People are not stupid. They find what works and stick to it. The primary motivation is usually self-care, not self-destruction.

Another driving force in the development of a harm reduction model was the recognition that traditional programs did not work for a large number of people, despite the AA slogan "Keep coming back: It works." The popular perception of the 12-Step programs as highly successful "treatment" is not borne out by the statistics on attendance or the research on relapse rates (Fox, 1993; Peele, 1991; Thombs, 1994).

The argument that some people are just not ready or not honest enough to get into recovery is put forward as a defense against what appear to be poor outcomes. Treatment outcomes should be analyzed according to many factors. Was the diagnosis correct? Was the treatment chosen with the diagnosis and the individual in mind? Was the therapist competent? And, of course, were there patient factors that contributed to the failure, such as poor attendance, lying, irregular medication compliance, lack of transportation or child care, racial or gender differences? Public health models are more likely to focus on issues of accessibility, needs assessment, and service delivery, including staffing patterns that reflect the community served.

The field of alcohol and drug treatment is languishing for several reasons. Funding for alternative theories or treatments is difficult to obtain. Much drug treatment funding is geared toward research into the biological aspects of addiction, and little disagreement has been allowed within the 12-Step community. *The Big Book* of Alcoholics Anonymous (1939/1976) is still the primary tool used. Mental health professionals have largely opted out of the drug treatment field, partly because many treatment programs refuse to use psychological approaches. As a result, the 12-Step recovery movement and the treatment centers that utilize its model are populated primarily by paraprofessional counselors who use the same methods that worked for their own recovery. The result is an experientially based, subjective approach, often rigidly applied to another person's problems (Thombs, 1994).

Harm reduction psychotherapy stresses the role of psychological problems in the development of the most serious drug use disorders. Psychodynamic theory and research point to significant problems with affect modulation and tolerance, deficits that make the person vulnerable to what for others may be difficult, but tolerable reactions to everyday life and to stressors.

Clinicians and researchers' recent attention to the dually diagnosed patient, one who has both significant psychiatric and substance use problems, is laudable. However, these patients have been around for the past 50 years, while both the mental health field and the chemical dependency field argued over who would care for them. Most often, these patients received no care and were referred to as "double trouble." Because this new clinical model views drug use as an adaptive mechanism, and drug abuse as a result of biopsychosocial forces, this distinction between psychological and drug use disorders is unnecessary. One can assume that all people use drugs for reasons, and furthermore, that those people who develop what Peele (1991) calls severe, *persistent addictions* are all dually diagnosed in the strictest sense of the term. Chapter 6 explores the clinical issues with this population in more depth.

Often, mental health professionals mistakenly ignore the physiological processes that accompany significant drug use, focusing only on the symptom aspects of the behavior. They are unaware of the development of functional autonomy, a process whereby chronic drug use becomes unmoored from its original psychological motivations and mechanisms, resulting in what the disease model would call "loss of control" and "progression" of the disease.

Disease model proponents also blind themselves to important physiological information. Because addiction is seen as unitary, the same for everybody, few distinctions are made between the physiological and psychological effects of different drugs. Alcohol is quite different in its effects within both the body and the psyche from stimulants such as cocaine or methamphetamine. Blurring these distinctions results in treatment that is too general and that may be completely inappropriate for a given individual.

Once the clinician recognizes the importance of these many factors in the development of substance use disorders, it becomes necessary to develop a comprehensive assessment protocol. Standard questions regarding the use, duration of use, and dosage are not sufficient to cover the myriad psychological, social, and physical dimensions of addiction. The approach that I have developed includes such an assessment, termed the Multidisciplinary Assessment Profile (MAP). This tool is described at length in Chapter 3.

# PART *II*

---

# *HARM REDUCTION PSYCHOTHERAPY IN ACTION*

# CHAPTER THREE

# *The Treatment Program: Assessment as Treatment*

## INTRODUCTION TO THE MULTIDISCIPLINARY ASSESSMENT PROFILE

Although clinical training in psychology has always emphasized the importance of doing a thorough assessment before developing a treatment plan, mental health professionals or chemical dependency specialists too often fail to conduct such an assessment. The resulting treatment obscures important individual differences, often causing poor retention of patients in treatment, lack of success, and recidivism rates that are common in chemical dependency treatment.

This chapter describes the Multidisciplinary Assessment Profile (MAP), a baseline tool for working with chemical dependency clients. The need for this profile, which I developed over years of clinical experience, is crucial for clients with more complex problems, especially dual- or multidiagnosed clients (people with concurrent psychiatric and/or medical disorders and substance abuse problems). Of course, in cases in which a client presents with a relatively straightforward alcohol or drug problem (i.e., no concurrent medical or psychiatric syndrome), it may not be necessary to conduct the full assessment described in this chapter. Among such clients might be young persons or those persons who respond to acute situational crises with an increase in drug or alcohol use. I present the details of a complex assessment here because many of the cases we see in day-to-day practice do in fact present with such complicating factors.

Central to a harm reduction psychotherapy model is the belief that what we typically refer to as assessment is, in actual practice, a phase of treatment that is integrated into the entire treatment process. The MAP is an assessment method that has three distinct and integrated functions: (1) the gathering of standard clinical and demographic data during the initial interviews; (2) techniques that increase the likelihood that such information will be honestly offered by the client; and (3) the development of a mutually honest and trusting working relationship that will form the foundation for any subsequent interactions between the client and therapist. Harm reduction psychotherapy relies on the development of a stable, therapeutic relationship to further the investigative and treatment process.

This chapter presents 12 areas of inquiry that constitute the MAP and details the important tasks to be accomplished during the clinical interviews. After each of the 12 sections, I present information from Joan's case history, introduced in Chapter 2. Details of her symptoms will help the reader see the practical applications of each of the assessment areas. Again, in this model, the assessment and treatment are usually concurrent. I have separated them only in order to examine each more closely and to provide the specific skills necessary for the implementation of a complex therapeutic process.

A comprehensive assessment includes information about the whole individual in addition to information about substance abuse behaviors. With many clients who self-refer because they are often experiencing distress about their substance use, these interviews can be more direct and detail-oriented. These clients may be either extremely informed about their drug use or relatively naive and dumbfounded when they find themselves in trouble.

Just as in psychotherapy for other disorders, working with the drug user requires that the clinician time questions and interventions with the state of the therapeutic relationship in mind. Other clients, particularly involuntary clients, are understandably more guarded and may appear initially uncooperative or resistant. The guidelines for motivational interviewing described here are absolutely necessary with persons in this population, since they have not yet agreed upon participation in treatment. Continuation of treatment relies primarily on the rapid establishment of a therapeutic alliance.

Even an initially motivated and cooperative client can be made to feel defensive in a therapeutic interview. In this model, the responsibility for lowering resistance is shared by client and therapist.

## MOTIVATIONAL INTERVIEWING

Some clinicians have recently reworked their understanding of the complex processes and motivations for change. Researchers also have made a major contribution to this newer understanding and have opened up the possibility of revolutionizing chemical dependency treatment through the use of a simple method termed motivational interviewing (Miller & Rollnick, 1991). Motivational interviewing is both a treatment strategy and a technique for interviewing clients. The word "interviewing" should be thought of in the same way that Sullivan (1954) used the term "the psychiatric interview," that is, as a prolonged inquiry that both gathers information and builds the therapeutic relationship. Information gathering per se is only a small part of the "interview." The development of a therapeutic relationship is of primary importance.

Efforts to assess a client's motivation or readiness for traditional chemical dependency treatment have usually relied on concepts such as "hitting bottom," which assumes that a person must experience serious negative consequences before he or she will be amenable to treatment. Resistance to treatment is also assumed to be an indicator of poor motivation. In the mental health field, failure to keep an appointment, arriving late, or spending the session talking about "peripheral" issues have been similarly construed. In both mental health and chemical dependency fields, clinical staff often feel little responsibility for increasing motivation, nor do they have much confidence in their ability to increase it. This passivity has caused many clients to reject treatment, with resulting poor retention and outcome.

Much chemical dependency literature also relies on the concepts of denial and lack of motivation for treatment to explain the difficulties of working with people with substance use disorders. In contrast, motivational interviewing is based on several assumptions that contrast with those traditionally used in chemical dependency work. Miller and Rollnick (1991) suggest that motivation is not a stable trait residing within the individual; rather, it is a flexible state existing within an interpersonal matrix. Motivation, viewed this way, suggests (as research asserts) that the therapist has a unique *ability* and *responsibility* to enhance a client's motivation for change. This is an inherently hopeful stance that requires clinicians to develop strategies for enhancing motivation.

Miller and Rollnick elaborate these strategies in two phases: (1) building the client's motivation to change, and (2) strengthening the client's commitment to change. The following is a summary of the techniques involved in the first stage of motivational interviewing.

1. *Express empathy*. Let the client know that you understand his or her wish to deal with a problem and that you appreciate both his or her efforts and the difficulty of the situation.

2. *Develop discrepancy*. Emphasize the client's expressed awareness of any drawbacks to his or her use of alcohol or drugs ("You are afraid that your smoking pot might be getting in the way of studying for the final exam").

3. *Avoid argumentation*. There is no right answer about a person's drug or alcohol use. You are trying to understand the *client's* perspective, not impose some external authority.

4. *Roll with resistance*. Ambivalence is normal and healthy, and resistance can be a sign of ego strength. You are not the boss. Do not put yourself in that position. Reflect back the *client's own ambivalence and confusions* about his or her drug use ("On the one hand, you feel that your drinking has gotten worse over the years, but you aren't at all convinced that you have to quit totally").

5. *Support self-efficacy*. Research consistently shows that a person who feels confident about his or her ability to make a change is much more likely to do so. What may sound to you like denial or false confidence is often felt by the client to be a *statement of faith in him- or herself* ("So, it sounds like even though you have been using cocaine every day, you feel pretty sure you can quit whenever you decide to").

These techniques reflect genuine respect for the client and a belief that, with help, the client can arrive at a responsible decision about addictive behaviors. No time line is suggested for developing motivation that leads to change. For some people, the process will be relatively quick, taking only a few sessions. Others may need a year or more before significant motivation is built. Clinicians trained in providing psychotherapy should not be surprised that chemical dependency treatment, even the first phase of such treatment, may be a long-term proposition.

The reader may recognize the techniques described as modifications of basic Rogerian methods, especially active and reflective listening. A major difference between Rogerian techniques and motivational interviewing is the clinical decision about which client statements should receive attention and reflection. Statements reflecting concern about drug use; any intention, direct or implicit, to change the drug use; and optimism about changing are considered *self-motivational statements* and are the main sources for reflection by the therapist. Eliciting and reflecting self-motivational statements is an art in which the therapist carefully chooses the client's own words and resists the urge to emphasize or punctuate with statements or feelings not originally articulated by the client. Such therapeutic overkill, which we often call interpretation, has no place in the early stages of motivational interviewing. Therapists are not attempting to educate or change clients, but to educate themselves about the clients, as well as reflecting back clients' own concerns about their own substance use.

Many strategies may be used to support these techniques. One is to ask open-ended questions that require a bit of thought—more than a "yes" or "no" answer. This encourages introspection and avoids the problems arising in an often adversarial question-and-answer interview format ("How do you see your work and your drug use fitting together?" rather than "Do you think your drug use is affecting your work?").

Still another strategy is to group communications into chunks that can be fed back to the client in shorter form. Summarizing the conversation as it progresses gives the therapist the opportunity to correct any misinterpretations and offers a chance for the client to elaborate further ("Let me see if I understand what you've said so far. On the one hand, your friends are concerned that you're drinking too much, but you don't think you drink any more than they do. On the other hand, you don't like getting hangovers, and that's been happening more lately. Have I left anything out?").

In clinical practice, the use of the motivational interviewing approach results in interaction that is honest, informative, and therapeutic. Patients feel respected and empowered, and therapists feel hopeful and *aligned with their patients,* not against them, and their problem behaviors. Once again, it is important to see addicts as people with problems rather than as problematic people.

## THE MULTIDISCIPLINARY ASSESSMENT PROFILE

The clinician's final assessment should reflect an understanding of many different dimensions of a person's personality. While the MAP is presented in a particular order that can be used to guide the interview process, the actual decisions about what information to gather at what point is a matter of the therapist's clinical judgment. For example, often, it is not wise to ask about specific drug use patterns early in treatment (the first two or three sessions) when it is obvious that the client is feeling either defensive or extremely ashamed of the drug use. In such a case, it is more important to develop rapport and communicate interest in the whole client, not just in his or her drug use. Treatment is based on the interplay of different factors that can be seen as the relative strengths and weaknesses of a particular client. The 12 listed components are described and then linked to one case in order to see how they present in a real person. We follow the client, Joan, through the entire assessment process.

1. *Stage of change*: Where the client fits in a motivational schema.
2. *Decisional balance*: The client's understanding of the benefits and consequences of his or her drug use.
3. *Type of drug(s) used*: Including frequency, amounts, patterns of use.
4. *Level of abuse or dependence*
   - Delineate the continuum of use → abuse → addiction.
   - Interactions of drug, set, and setting.
   - Known or presumed negative biopsychosocial consequences (especially relating to interpersonal problems,

HIV and other medical disorders, psychiatric problems, pregnancy, etc.).
- Client's level of control over use.

5. *Prescribed medications*: Current and past prescribed medicines, including patterns of compliance.
6. *Past treatment history*: A history of the client's attempts to stop or reduce substance use, including:
   - Specific efforts that helped or hindered.
   - Subjective experience of past treatment or attempts to quit or reduce substance use.
7. *Support system.* Helpful, harmful, or absent?
8. *Self-efficacy*: The client's degree of confidence in ability to control or to make changes in his or her own life, including drug use.
9. *Psychiatric diagnosis*: Psychosocial history, DSM-IV diagnosis, and observational and patient's subjective statement about the impact of drug use on mental disorder, for example, does substance use exacerbate problems, is it helpful for self-medication, or both?
10. *Client's stated goal(s)*: Including type(s) of treatment desired as well as types of treatment rejected.
11. *Therapist's stated goal(s)*: Including rationale for treatment goals.
12. *Developmental grid*: Outline of key events and personality traits that will be used to guide treatment.

Data may be gathered from many sources, including the following:

- Standard psychiatric interviews.
- Laboratory tests for general organ/system functioning, immune system, toxicology screenings, neurological exam, nutritional status, and so on.
- Specific assessment tools for various drug problems, such as the *Alcohol Use Inventory* (AUI-R; Horn, Wanberg, & Foster, 1987), or the *Addiction Severity Index* (McLellan, Luborsky, Woody, & O'Brien, 1980).
- Psychological testing to rule out underlying psychosis.
- Special attention to Axis II symptomatology/patterns.

Each of the following sections suggests relevant questions to be asked and answered. The results of this assessment will be the foundation for treatment decisions about primary focus, goals, matching, intensity, and technique. After a brief reintroduction to the case mentioned in Chapter 2 (Joan), this chapter offers detailed information regarding each section of the assessment profile, followed by the application of the assessment technique with Joan.

## Case History

Joan came to therapy because of a recent breakup with a girlfriend. She felt depressed, anxious, and hopeless about ever achieving a long- term relationship. At 27 years of age, Joan had had a series of very short- term relationships, none lasting longer than a few months. She described a pattern of becoming intensely attached to another woman and very quickly becoming insecure and jealous. She acted out these feelings by making "scenes" in public, thus humiliating her girlfriend by subjecting her to increasingly unrealistic demands for attention and reassurance. The girlfriend, feeling suffocated, embarrassed, and angry, would break up with Joan with little discussion. Only reluctantly did Joan talk about her awareness of the origins of her jealous and insecure feelings. She made it clear that her childhood was difficult and that she did not particularly want to dwell on the past.

Almost as an aside, Joan gave me information about her drug and alcohol use (as noted in Chapter 2). Given the story she told, it is no wonder that it was difficult for me to maintain an open and encouraging manner. My impulse was to react with worry and act out my need to fix her quickly. Joan was using large quantities of alcohol, at least seven to nine drinks per day, every day. She supplemented this by snorting and at times injecting powder cocaine. She also took large amounts of a narcotic painkiller that was being prescribed by her orthopedist for severe hip pain. While somewhat defensive when talking about her drug use, she offered the information without my asking, indicating to me that she was at least aware that *I* would consider it important information even if she did not label it as such.

Joan gave a brief family history during the first session. She and her older brother were born and raised in a rural area in South Dakota. Her parents died in a car accident when she was 5, and Joan and her brother were sent to live in an orphanage where they were both physically and sexually abused. Joan's brother committed suicide in the orphanage when he was 12 years old, and she was released to the care of an elderly female relative shortly after that, when she was 11. This mother figure was kind to her, and the two of them often sat around drinking sherry and singing songs, an activity that did not seem odd to Joan at the time.

Despite such a difficult beginning, Joan managed to complete her education and, at the time of intake, had been working as a chemical research assistant in the same lab for more than 5 years. She was well liked and given a lot of responsibility, which she enjoyed. She stated that no one at work knew what a "mess" she was, and she intended to keep it that way.

At this point, I discuss each part of the assessment in more detail, using the case of Joan to illustrate the ideas that can then be applied to other patients.

## Stages of Change

Any time people wish to make a change in their lives, whether it involves a complex series of decisions, like switching jobs, or a relatively straightforward choice, like quitting smoking, they go through several *stages of change*. Addictive behaviors are often the target of such decisions and attempts to change. In psychotherapy, behavior change is the overt result of many internal and external factors. Changing drug use is essentially the same internal and external process despite the fact that people tend to see it as only an overt behavior. Researchers have recently focused specifically on how behavior change takes place within persons. Not surprisingly, they found that people tend to go through the same process and stages when trying to change drug or alcohol use as they do when deciding to change jobs or start an exercise program (Prochaska, DiClemente, & Norcross, 1992).

Important concepts in this theory of the stages of change include the fluidity of change and the importance of self-efficacy in both the initiation and maintenance of change. Clinical assessment of the client's place along the continuum of change provides a broader view of the person and creates possibilities for the development of interventions specific to the individual at a particular point in the treatment process. Thus, clinical interventions can be designed to match the client's current stage of change and assist in the *natural process* of changing.

## Stage 1: Precontemplation

This stage may be termed the "Who, me?" stage. Clients either do not identify drug use as a problem or only express passive wishes that things were different. No intention to change exists at this point, at least not in the near future. This stance is often characterized by others as denial, but is actually only an indication of a lack of information. Other people in clients' lives may fervently wish for change and may pressure them into seeking treatment. In this case, the persons making the referral are in a different stage of change than the clients. The therapist who is aware of this difference can prevent common pitfalls in therapeutic encounters, such as assuming that clients want to change and confronting them if they do not. The clinician should realize that while some clients may not identify their substance use as a problem, they may still be willing to talk about other problems in their life. Allowing clients to do so may create an atmosphere for some form of treatment that can begin immediately. Strategic therapists might refer to this type of person as a "visitor" for substance abuse treatment, but a "customer" for working on stress reduction (Berg & Miller, 1992). It is important to keep in mind that the development of a working relationship does not necessarily begin with the sharing of common goals. Rather, it is part of the work to establish a therapeutic agenda that both client and therapist can work toward together.

## Stage 2: Contemplation

During this stage, clients more readily acknowledge a problem and that they might want to do something about it. This stage can be seen as the "Yes, but" stage ("Sure I drink too much sometimes, but I can quit whenever I want to"). Another typical statement might be "I'd like to quit smoking cigarettes, but I'm under a lot of stress right now." Such people are actively (if not altogether consciously) assessing the pros and cons of their behavior along with the benefits and risks of change. The therapist's job is to encourage such ambivalence rather than label it as resistance or denial. The intrapsychic process is one of raising to consciousness both sides of the natural ambivalence that people feel when confronted with uncomfortable evidence. Premature settling on either side of the ambivalence about drug use is a common cause of treatment failure and relapse. Specific clinical interventions with people at this stage will be covered in the next section on the "decisional balance."

## Stage 3: Preparation

At this stage, people intend to make a change and are beginning to establish behavioral criteria for that change. They may already have reduced the amount or frequency of substance use, or intend to do so soon (usually within 1 month). While clients may not have decided on the exact nature of their goal (e.g., abstinence or moderation), they are exhibiting behaviors that point to change. A classic example is the person who abuses alcohol. This individual often decides to switch from distilled spirits ("hard liquor") to beer in an attempt to cut down on consumption. Clinicians often see this plan as a sign of denial and resistance rather than what it often is, an honest attempt to change a problem behavior while hoping that the change will not have to be too drastic. This wish is present in most people who are struggling with changing a behavior that is patterned and that gives them at least some satisfaction. Buying "low fat" cookies and cakes is an obvious example of attempting to make a change that is less radical than giving up sweets altogether. Clinicians are often blind to the similarities between people who use drugs and people who engage in other types of behaviors labeled as problems. While we would never fault a person who wants to keep chocolate in his diet, we are suspicious of someone who wants to keep drinking at a lower level, or who wants to smoke marijuana on occasion. (The fact is, most people can eat chocolate and not develop serious problems. On the other hand, some people eat too much and gain extra weight or put themselves at risk for diabetes. What we often fail to realize is that most people who drink or use marijuana *also do so* with little harm. Some, do, however, develop problems associated with such drug use.)

## Stage 4: Action

Behavior changes become evident at this stage. The person commits much time and effort to deciding on the details of the process (when to start the change, how much to change, supports necessary, etc.), and other people also recognize these attempts. A specific criterion has also been established, such as quitting drinking completely, or, in the case of weight control, exercising for 20 minutes per day. From this point on, clients have made a promise to themselves and have an external measure of success or failure, which, in turn combine to make them very vulnerable to narcissistic injury if they "backslide" or "slip up." Then, having broken a promise to themselves, and maybe to others as well, they are frightened and ashamed of the failure. The psychodynamic reactions to relapse and specific interventions to deal with this phenomenon are covered in the section on relapse prevention.

### Stage 5: Maintenance

This stage is an extended one in which persons learn new behaviors and coping strategies to maintain the change they have achieved. New relationship patterns are developed, and clients spend quite a bit of time and psychic energy practicing specific coping skills, such as distraction or drink refusal. Relapse prevention becomes a primary focus. Six months with no relapse is generally viewed as the time period required to consider a person in the maintenance stage. This stage may last for an extended period of time and, for some, may be considered a lifetime proposition.

### Relapse

Relapse, though not a stage of change, is an integral component of the change process. Most people who modify their behavior do not maintain that change the first time they try. Relapse is the rule, not the exception, when changing any habit, including drug or alcohol use. People learn important things during and after relapse, and gain experience with risk situations for the first time. For example, a person who has abstained from alcohol for 6 months but drinks at an open bar at a wedding now knows he may easily be able to resist *buying* a drink but has not learned how to resist a *free* one.

During relapse, persons revert back to a previous stage of change, often precontemplation (Stage 1). The vast majority of people cycle back to the contemplation and preparation stages and begin again to implement action. Clients are particularly vulnerable during relapse, again partly because of the narcissistic injury experienced. Often, they have been taught that relapses are inevitable, dangerous, and damaging, creating a self-fulfilling prophecy in which clients withdraw from treatment because they feel the inevitability of disastrous consequences during relapse. The therapist must defuse such fears prior to relapse, teach specific skills to help people stop any "sliding" once a slip has occurred, and above all, create an atmosphere of acceptance of clients and confidence in their ability to succeed even if they do relapse. Most importantly, the therapist must develop a relationship with clients that reflects tolerance of the shifts and delays that accompany any major life change.

## Stage 6: Termination

There is a popular idea that recovery from drug or alcohol abuse is a lifelong process; the actual research on change takes a surprising turn. People do, in fact, reach a point in time where the behavior no longer threatens to intrude on daily life. After a certain amount of time, a client does not need to be careful of situations or people that were once associated with the behavior. Avoiding people, places, and things is not forever essential for the person to maintain his or her goal, whether it be to avoid alcohol, or to have only one cookie when a plateful is offered. Assuming that termination will occur, the therapist can assess progress in ways similar to assessment of progress in any psychotherapy. Symptom reduction or elimination, increased performance and satisfaction with work and relationships, and improved physical health are indicators that the person's work is near finished. Rather than warn the patient regarding the continuing dangers of relapse into drug addiction, the therapist can join with the patient in an evaluation and a celebration of change.

\*　　　\*　　　\*

Joan presented a confusing picture in terms of both her present position in the stages of change and her previous stance toward change. In the past, she had tried to quit using drugs and alcohol several times with little or no success. This indicated that Joan, at some point, had been through the different stages of contemplation, preparation, and action.

Lately, however, it appeared that she might have been at the stage of precontemplation again, because she did not identify her drug use during intake as a significant part of her presenting problems. She was not, however, totally unwilling to entertain the possibility that certain drug use behaviors might be problematic, specifically, her use of cocaine and alcohol. Joan adamantly refused to consider changing her use of prescription narcotics because she saw them as medically, rather than psychologically, necessary. So Joan was in different stages with different substances.

### Stages of Change Summary for Joan

- Stage 1: Precontemplation
  Narcotics: Joan has no intention of changing this behavior and does not see any negative consequences associated with her narcotic use.
- Stages 1 and 2: Precontemplation and contemplation
  Cocaine, alcohol, and marijuana: Joan is willing to entertain the possibility that some of these drugs may cause problems some of the time, but she has not articulated specific examples.

With this type of profile, the clinician has to be careful to follow the client as she tells the story of her difficulties, rather than assume to know the consequences of her drug use. She is clearly in distress, wants some relief, and has come to therapy expecting help. Despite her history, which would alert any clinician to the presence of significant psychopathology, Joan's strengths must also be noted and respected. She has asked for specific help with relationship problems and it would be wise to focus on her agenda.

### Decisional Balance

The next phase of the assessment process is a technique called the *decisional balance* (Janis & Mann, 1977). Joan's case highlights the importance of this area of assessment. The decisional balance is a conceptual, behavioral, and affective "display" of the ambivalence a person feels about her substance use. Many clinicians view this ambivalence as either a source of potent resistance or a denial of problems, either of which foretells treatment failure. A more productive way of understanding this is to acknowledge that people began to use drugs for adaptive reasons, for example, a client began to use psychoactive agents to manage feelings of sadness or anger, or to enhance social interactions. Despite the fact that considerable negative consequences may have accrued over time, these original (positive) adaptive reasons for substance use persist in the unconscious life of even the most "motivated" client. What this means in terms of assessment is that most people retain significant conscious or unconscious ambivalence about their drug or alcohol use, no matter what their stage of change when they first present. In other words, the person who is unsure whether or not a certain drug use pattern is a problem may not be that different psychologically from the person who comes in "ready to change" or already in the "action" stage.

While the client's ambivalence is most obvious during the contemplation stage, it is operative in all stages. It is tempting to treat the person in the action stage with robust reinforcement about the negative effects of substance use and the positive effects of change. Reinforcing a client to fear relapse is one technique often used. However, *this may be one of the primary reasons for relapse* in people in early recovery, because fear undermines their sense of confidence or self-efficacy and thus increases the chances of failure. Similarly, it is tempting to treat clients in the contemplation stage by confronting obvious negative consequences they may be denying. Both approaches ignore or minimize any powerful, positive reason(s) for clients' continued substance use. The systematic use of the decisional balance communicates the therapist's acceptance of patients' ambivalence while reminding the therapist of the need to work on many different levels at once. While initially used as an assessment tool by the therapist, the decisional balance will form a cornerstone for ongoing treatment with clients.

There are several ways to construct a decisional balance worksheet as an assessment tool. However, it is preferable to begin with a worksheet that is not too conceptually complex. People who are using drugs, or who have recently stopped, may have occult (hidden) cognitive problems even when they are not obviously impaired. Abstract reasoning is often diminished in clients whose drug use includes heavy alcohol intake or excessive use of tranquilizers. Paranoid thinking may be evident in long-term stimulant users. For these reasons it is best to avoid complex cognitive tasks until the therapist knows the clients better and has assessed cognitive functions.

To begin, the therapist takes a sheet of blank paper and divides it into two halves (see Figure 3.1).

*Typical Questions to Begin the Process*
- "You've said you want to quit drinking. What do you think will be good for you if you do quit?"
- "What positive things do you expect to gain?"
- "On the other hand, can you imagine what might be the downside of quitting? What might not be so good for you?"

*Or one might ask the following questions:*
- "What have you noticed about your drug use that you like?"
- "How do you think the amount of speed you're using may affect your sleep problems?"

CHANGE MY DRINKING/DRUG USE

Pros                                                        Cons

_ _ _ _ _ _ _ _ _ _ _ _ _ _ _ _ _ _ _ _ _ _ _ _ _ _ _ _

CONTINUE USING THE WAY I AM NOW

Pros                                                        Cons

FIGURE 3.1. The Decisional Balance Worksheet.

The therapist has the client record his or her responses in the top section of the worksheet or uses a flip chart. If the client cannot produce responses, the therapist uses what information he or she already has from the client's statements to fill in the worksheet, then asks if the statements fit the client's beliefs and feelings. This gives the therapist an opportunity to communicate your empathic understanding of what the patient has previously related. It also gives the client a chance to correct any misconceptions. If the therapist encounters denial or resistance to statements, it is possible that he or she has either overstated the client's feelings or hit on a sensitive area that needs to be explored more at a later time. When this difficulty occurs, it is imperative not to argue with the client or attempt to "clarify" the specific words. The therapist simply says that he or she has misunderstood and asks the client to repeat his or her thoughts and feelings. These techniques of motivational interviewing will help guide the therapist through the delicate process of information gathering when the client is feeling defensive or seems reluctant to share details.

It is interesting to note that if a therapist "misquotes" the client while attempting to help articulate pros and cons of drug use, he will probably revert to a previous stage of change. This clearly indicates a resistance based on felt misunderstanding and could cause a rupture of the fragile therapeutic alliance that has been building. The therapist's task then shifts from information gathering to alliance building, a shift that can be expected to happen frequently throughout the assessment (and perhaps the treatment) phase.

As mentioned before, the decisional balance is both an assessment tool and an ongoing instrument for treatment and progress review. The client may not, at first, be able to articulate pros and cons relevant to his substance use, especially if he is in acute distress, in the action stage, or involuntarily committed for treatment. In these instances, the therapist should be prepared to initiate and perhaps actually do the bulk of the initial work.

This method of conceptualizing the decisional balance process places responsibility on the therapist to conduct the interview in a way that builds rapport and elicits cooperation. Although the patient has a concurrent responsibility, he may be incapable of full participation in the process because of the very problems that brought him into treatment or because of the stigma attached to his drug use.

*          *          *

Joan was reluctant to take the time to fill in the decisional balance worksheet. She thought it took up therapy time that she wanted to use to focus on relationship problems. After my questioning led Joan to make a connection between her alcohol use and fighting with her girlfriend, we agreed to use part of her session as she wished and part to work specifically on her alcohol use. This agreement acknowledged the client as both the "customer," who was in the preparation stage for relationship change, and the "visitor," who was in the contemplation stage regarding her drug use. Joan's decisional balance Worksheet looked like Figure 3.2 when we were through filling it out. The process took about 10 weeks. For the sake of brevity, I have condensed separate decisional balance worksheets for each specific drug into one summary sheet.

It is apparent from this early list that Joan was very ambivalent about changing her drug use and saw only a few potent reasons to do so. Recognizing this allows the clinician to focus treatment on identifying more reasons to change rather than reasons to stay the same. This identification could be done directly or by using material Joan has talked about regarding her relationship problems. For example, the therapist might want to ask, "How would drinking affect your relationship?" or "How do you think alcohol affected the fight you and your girlfriend had yesterday?" It is important to ask open-

### CHANGE MY DRINKING/DRUG USE

| Pros | Cons |
|---|---|
| I'd save money. | I'd have trouble sleeping |
| I wouldn't have hangovers. | I couldn't hang out in bars with my friends. |
| I wouldn't hurt my veins/arms. | My hip would hurt all the time. |
| Maybe I wouldn't be as moody. | I'd get suicidal. |

### CONTINUE USING THE WAY I AM NOW

| Pros | Cons |
|---|---|
| No withdrawal period. | Might overdose. |
| Nothing would have to change. | Might lose my job. |
| I wouldn't feel lonely. | |

FIGURE 3.2. Joan's decisional balance worksheet.

ended questions rather than simple "yes–no" questions. Closed questions often cause defensiveness and tend to end discussion, with little information gained.

At first glance, it might seem that the two main categories, "change," and "keep the same" are identical. With cognitively impaired or emotionally restricted patients, the subtle differences may go unnoticed. When this is the case, the therapist fills in the decisional balance worksheet using only half of the paper, leaving more complex associations until a later time.

## Type of Drugs Used

An inventory of *types of drugs used* should be conducted with the realization that some patterns of alcohol or drug use may fall into the realm of recreational or nonpathological use. Despite current cultural beliefs and biases, many people do, in fact, use legal and illegal drugs in ways that do not constitute abuse, as no apparent harm results from these behaviors. Some may argue that any use of illicit drugs is abuse since it entails the risk of arrest. While this is technically true, it is of little use clinically when a therapist deals with a patient who uses cocaine a few times a month when he goes out dancing. There is probably no way to convince such a person that he is suffering from drug abuse without rupturing the therapeutic alliance.

While clinicians must gather specific, historical information about the age of the patient at the time of first substance use, patterns of use, and changes in use over time, it is not necessary, or even prudent, to focus on this information in the first session or two. Clinicians in the field offer varying perspectives regarding the timing of taking a drug history. Using the stages of change as a guide, it would not be desirable to begin such a detailed inquiry with a client who is in the precontemplation stage, and perhaps not even in the contemplation stage, when his motivation is fluid. Nor would a detailed drug history fit with a psychotherapy perspective in which one would hope to bring out subtle dynamics in the person's patterns. Doing so redirects the client's attention away from the complex psychosocial aspects of his drug use in favor of a purely historical rendering of facts and details (Mark & Faude, 1997), and inevitably set a tone for the therapy that may be difficult to redirect. It is a safer strategy to wait until information of a more psychological nature emerges, tie it to possible links with substance use, and only later, when the patient is sure that the therapist is truly interested in *all* of him, ask for specific details to fill out the assessment.

The clinician should also be aware that for some people, substance use patterns may temporarily become problematic due to psychosocial stressors at development milestones or during crises. While such changes in substance use may require brief intervention, they should not be construed as evidence of a developing chronic disorder. Education and supportive counseling are often enough to return the person to nonpathological substance use patterns, especially with adolescents and young adults. Research indicates that most serious consequences of substance abuse do not occur until the person's drug use has continued into adulthood (see Brunswick et al., 1992), so early intervention techniques need *not* presume that the patient is on a deteriorating course. This type of drug misuse is analogous to gaining 5 or 10 pounds over a long holiday or vacation. This weight gain, although the result of overindulgence in food and perhaps detrimental to one's health if continued over the long run, should not be construed as an eating disorder. Similarly, a few experiences of heavy drinking do not make one an alcoholic.

Many clinicians and agencies develop their own substance use history sheets, which may be a simple form that asks questions about specific substances used, client's age at first use, frequency, amounts, and/or current pattern. Others may prefer letting clients identify verbally the specific drugs they have used rather than check off from a list of all types of substances on a form. The primary goal is to gather historical information about specific substances used, in what quantities, by what route of administration, and in what patterns over a period of time. However, it is preferable, if possible, to avoid the use of checklists at the beginning of treatment. Since use of a drug history checklist isolates this piece of information gathering from the direct therapeutic relationship, it may result in incomplete or inaccurate information if the relationship has not yet developed enough mutual trust. Of course, some insurance companies require that a full drug and alcohol assessment be done quickly, often in the first session. In these cases, the therapist might have the patient fill out the necessary questions in the waiting room and turn them in rather than conduct a question-and-answer interview.

One problem that often occurs during assessment is that most therapists have not been trained in specific interviewing techniques that evoke important substance use information. Quite often, the person using the drug knows much more about it than the clinician. On the other hand, some substance users have significant misinformation that might obscure their issues. While clinicians need a working knowledge of major substances in order to ask detailed questions, they also should be willing to ask clients to educate them about substances and how they are used. Appendix A offers a brief description of the major groups of drugs that are often abused, as well as typical routes of administration, short-term effects of intoxication, and long-term medical consequences of abuse. This information is of great use to the clinician who is relatively naive about drugs.

Before returning to the case example, I want to emphasize the importance of getting an *accurate* assessment of the quantity of alcohol or drugs that the person is using. This information will determine how quickly the person may be able to quit or cut down use and whether medical intervention might be necessary. In addition, the amount that persons actually use is often a mystery to them. This is especially the case with alcohol. Raising the level of consciousness regarding the quantity used will often increase motivation for change. With drugs in pill form, consulting a pharmacist or a reference book such as the *Physicians' Desk Reference* (Medical Economics Co., 1998) may be useful. In the case of drugs that are generally in powder form and are either smoked, injected, or snorted, it may be more difficult to ascertain the quantity ingested. With these drugs, it is probably more important to understand the client's terminology regarding a standard dose, and determine amounts from that vantage point. For example, a person may say that she smokes heroin by putting it in a cigarette. The easiest way for a therapist to determine the relative dose is to ask how much of a balloon or other container of heroin the person uses per cigarette. On the other hand, the person injecting speed will usually know the amount (one to five grams per day) but will have no idea of the potency. Only alcohol and pharmaceutical pills allow us to measure precisely the amount of drug being ingested. It is imperative that clinicians accurately assess the *amount* of pure alcohol that a patient drinks. For instance, a large tumbler of wine may easily equal two or three reported "drinks"! Without accurate information, progress toward a goal other than abstinence is impossible to measure. Inaba, Cohen, and Holstein (1997) condense this information as follows:

One drink (1 oz. of pure alcohol) is equal to:
1 can (12 oz.) of regular beer
7 oz. of malt liquor
5 oz. of wine
10 oz. of wine cooler
1.5 oz. of 85-proof distilled spirits, including brandy

\*      \*      \*

Clinical inquiry resulted in the following information.

- *ETOH* (alcohol). Use started at age 6, when Joan would visit her grandmother. She used no alcohol from ages 7–11, while she was in an orphanage. Joan began drinking again with her grandmother at age 11, and by age 13, she was drinking episodically and heavily (five to ten drinks per episode). Current use equals five to eight drinks per day, nearly every day.
- *Marijuana.* Joan began smoking pot with friends at age 14. Since then, regular, moderate use involves one joint, three times per week.
- *Cocaine.* Joan first used at age 21. She snorted powdered cocaine one or two times weekly until the past year. Joan now uses daily, approximately one-fourth to one-half gram. She also occasionally injects cocaine intravenously, using up to a full gram at one time. She injects as often as once per week, but usually once per monthly.
- *Prescription narcotics.* Joan began using prescribed Vicodin (oxycodone with aspirin) for a serious hip disorder 3 years ago. She continues to use six to eight pills per day (a total of 30–40 mg), and sometimes uses Darvon (propoxyphene) instead. This amount of Vicodin, while perhaps within acceptable limits for severe pain, is being used in lieu of treatments that might reduce the pain (surgery and lifestyle changes). Significantly, she is mixing this amount of narcotics with heavy doses of alcohol as well.
- *Over-the-counter drugs (OTCs).* None.

### Level of Abuse or Dependence

It is important to keep in mind certain clinical data and diagnostic schemas when evaluating the nature of a person's drug use. The fourth edition of the *Diagnostic and Statistical Manual of Mental Disorders* (DSM-IV; American Psychiatric Association, 1994) lists criteria that include significant psychological and behavioral symptoms as well as patterns of actual drug use. *Substance abuse* is defined by a "maladaptive pattern" of drug or alcohol use that results in "significant adverse consequences" (p. 182). People with a substance abuse disorder continue to use drugs or alcohol despite suffering harm to themselves. The diagnosis of *substance dependence*, on the other hand, requires that there be both continued use despite negative consequences, and the presence of other symptoms that reflect a compulsive behavioral, cognitive, and physical pattern. Repetitive use often causes tolerance to the effects of the drug as well as a withdrawal syndrome upon abrupt discontinuation. Tolerance and withdrawal are not sufficient to make the diagnosis, however. There must be a clear cluster of symptoms that show that the substance use is occurring without the person's full control, indicated by attempts to quit or cut down, excessive attention paid to the drug or alcohol use to the detriment of other activities, a general curtailment of occupational or social roles, or physical problems associated with the drug or alcohol use (p. 181). Note that DSM-IV terminology often confuses clinicians and the public, who are more used to the term *addiction* to refer to compulsive patterns of drug use, often reserving the term *dependence* to mean physiological dependence. In this book, the terms *dependence* and *addiction* are used interchangeably, much as they are in clinical practice.

DSM-IV (American Psychiatric Association, 1994) has given clinicians a psychobiologically based criterion for diagnosis, but it does not make clear that there is in fact a continuum of drug use. It is important to understand this continuum for both assessment purposes and treatment. I have combined the definitions from several authors (e.g., Peele, 1991; Schuckit, 1989). Seven types of drug use are described. This continuum of use is not linear; that is, a person may move among these levels or stay in one for most of his or her life. It is not generally the case that most people in the first three levels develop abuse problems. Persons with abuse or dependence are generally at higher risk of developing long-lasting problems, but, again, this is not as common as popularly believed. In addition, the interacting effects of drug, set, and setting influence the level of addiction.

*The Continuum of Use*

1. *Experimentation.* The person tries a drug out of curiosity when it is available and has relatively few exposures to the drug.

2. *Social/recreational.* The drug is used for its specific effect but a pattern has not been established.

3. *Habituation.* A pattern of use has been established, but no problems occur, such as TGIF parties, snorting one-half gram of cocaine on weekends with friends while dancing, having two cups of coffee every morning, or drinking two glasses of wine each night with dinner. (*Note.* This type of alcohol use is controversial in the United States today. Many people see *any* regular use of a substance as problematic, an indication of an addictive attachment. Other people allow that regular social use of alcohol may not be a problem but consider any use of illicit drugs to be addictive in nature.)

4. *Abuse.* A person continues use despite negative consequences. As mentioned earlier, there is controversy about whether one should label the use of any illicit (illegal) substance as use rather than abuse. Some people consider use of a drug like cocaine, which could result in serious legal harm, to constitute enough risk to call it abuse. The term "abuse" clearly has no consensual definition in the profession. However, those who would define all use of illegal drugs as abuse miss the fundamental concepts that are important in diagnosis and treatment and are not differentiating between the harm cause by one drug versus another (or the harm caused by the legal sanctions themselves). They also ignore the fact that the legal status of a particular drug is a sociocultural phenomenon that has little to do with the drug itself (cigarettes are legal, as is alcohol, but both often cause significantly more medical problems than do marijuana or high-grade heroin). Automatically equating all drug use with abuse results in the contradictions and confusion that permeate the drug treatment field. For example, in disease model programs, a recovering alcoholic who sometimes smokes marijuana is said to be abusing marijuana because the program calls for abstinence from all psychoactive drugs. An exception is usually made for other, more socially acceptable psychoactive drugs such as nicotine and caffeine, however, making the distinction one of limited value for diagnosis and treatment.

5. *Dependence (addiction).* Abuse + compulsion + relapse potential. There is little agreement about the use of the term *depend-*

*ence* in the field, despite the DSM-IV definition. A person is labeled dependent when he has all the behavioral and cognitive symptoms of abuse to a more intense degree and is likely to resume destructive use of the drug or alcohol after a period of abstinence.

6. *Physiological dependence.* There is clear evidence of tissue and cellular accommodation. The person needs to use more of the drug to get the same effect (tolerance) and experiences a characteristic pattern of negative physical symptoms when the drug is stopped (withdrawal).

7. *Persistent addiction* (Peele, 1991). This is a term used to describe people who, after having developed an addiction, fail to change it significantly, with resulting deterioration. The pattern of use may be chaotic or maintenance. In the view of many people, addictions are by definition persistent; however, research shows that many people do change their destructive patterns of abuse or addiction without the help of professionals (Peele, 1991; Sobell, Cunningham, & Sobell, 1996). Peele (1991) refers to this *spontaneous recovery* as a process of *maturing out* (pp. 56–60). Many people manage to change their addictive patterns as they face adult responsibilities, lose adult rewards, or develop values that compete with the addiction. People who develop persistent addictions tend to be those with the most serious emotional, economic, or social difficulties. The pharmacology of the particular drug, while perhaps the cause of many negative consequences, is often less important for treatment purposes than is the emotional health of the person. These people consistently relapse after treatment. They are often poor, nonwhite, or otherwise marginalized (by mental illness, for example).

## Drug, Set, and Setting

The continuum of use is one way of assessing a person's relationship to drugs and alcohol. In order to create a more dynamic picture, however, it is useful to assess drug use patterns by identifying three interrelated factors: *drug* (substance), *set* (person), and *setting* (environment) (Zinberg, 1984). *Drug* refers to a number of factors related to the substance itself: its specific pharmacology and formulation, what is used to cut it, and the route of administration. We tend to think that it is the drug chemistry itself that has the greatest impact in creating addiction. But drug use is a function of a relationship. In fact, it is often the set or the setting in which a drug is used that de-termines the effect one gets from a drug. *Set* refers to the person us-ing the drug, and includes the motivation for using, the person's ex-pectation of the effect of the drug, the person's unique personality traits and psychodynamics, and whatever coping deficits the person may possess. *Setting* refers to a number of factors: a person's envi-ronment (and stressors), where the person uses and whether alone or with others (how at ease or rushed the person feels, for example, to take the dose with care); the legality of the substance used; and soci-etal attitudes toward the drug. Culture plays an important part in the setting as well. It is important to understand the cultural values and rituals with which the client was raised, and how the current culture either reflects the original milieu or is different or in conflict with it. The person may be part of a specific drug culture that has its own unique set of values and standards.

These three interrelated factors—drug, set, and setting—combine to create unique experiences for different people who may be using the same drug in the same quantity. Marijuana, LSD, and heroin are three drugs that are particularly set and setting dependent. The marijuana or LSD experience is responsive to the mood and expectations of the user and the safety and congeniality of the setting in which the drug is used. Some people report varying experiences with the same drug at different times. Heroin overdose is more likely in unfamiliar surroundings. This is true for people as well as animals in studies. Speculation is that a fa-miliar drug-use environment cues the user to undergo physiological preparation for the onset of the drug (Kuhn, Swartzwelder, & Wilson, 1998) In the absence of such automatic preparation, the body is more vulnerable to the drug's effects, including respiratory depression. These are the most dramatic examples of how set and setting affect the drug experience. Planned interventions that specifically target these individ-ual dynamics make the treatment more likely to be successful. Needless to say, the therapist must be both skilled at eliciting the details of a per-son's drug experience and comfortable hearing details that may be shocking or aversive.

*      *      *

Joan had consistently high levels of dependence on alcohol, nar-cotics, and cocaine. She presumably had a physiological dependence on both narcotics and alcohol (because of her daily high-dosage use). It is unclear whether she was physically dependent on the cocaine, as more information regarding withdrawal phenomena was needed. Surprisingly, given her pattern with other drugs, Joan showed only moderate, nonproblematic use of marijuana. She felt significant emotional distress and exhibited impaired social functioning, although her ability to continue working remained surprisingly intact. Joan did not, however, link her distress directly to her drug use. She was more likely to think that alcohol and shooting cocaine are the result of problems in her life. In fact, there was no clear evidence that her drug use caused negative effects in her life. I assume that continual use of so many substances in such quantities must have had something to do with her chronic relationship problems, but she gave me no direct evidence to back up my assumption.

Joan exhibited moderate loss of control with alcohol and cocaine, although one might speculate that her control was actually much more tenuous than the term "moderate" implies. Because she made no attempt to cut down, however, it is hard to say whether she was totally "out of control." She also experienced significant and increasing tolerance, but only to alcohol. Since alcohol and narcotics are mildly cross-tolerant, this probably allowed her to keep her prescription narcotic use steady. She also reported using prescription narcotics only to manage physical pain, not to deal with stress. She used alcohol socially as a way to enhance interactions, but she also used alone in order to reduce anxiety or to counter the effects of cocaine. In addition, Joan seemed to snort powder cocaine under very different circumstances than those under which she injected it. The effects of drug, set, and setting were present but not yet understood at this point in the assessment.

## Prescribed Medications

Clients commonly present one set of problems with alcohol or drugs but seem unaware of other problematic substance use related to *prescribed medications*. Currently, prescribed medications might include asthma medications, anti-inflammatory drugs (nonsteroidal anti-inflammatory drugs [NSAIDs] such as Motrin, etc.), or antidepressants (Prozac or Wellbutrin), for example. Clients might also be using one or more over-the-counter drugs (OTCs) as well, such as

Contac, Advil, or Benadryl. Prescription and OTC medications all have potential interactions that could cause physical or psychological symptoms. Many contain either stimulant or depressant ingredients.

In addition to specific prescription medications, the therapist needs to establish the client's pattern of compliance with the physician's directions for prescription medication use. For instance, when prescribed antibiotics, does the client take a full course or stop after only a few days? Or does the client take too many or too few pills of the medication? This information can give the therapist insight into characterological as well as pharmacological effects of prescription medications on the client's behaviors.

The use of holistic preparations such as vitamins, homeopathic remedies, or herbal preparations is also important to ascertain. Many holistic preparations contain active ingredients that may in themselves cause problems or interact with other drugs being used. A good example of a holistic preparation would be use of ginseng products (which generate high energy levels) by a person who also drinks lots of coffee and abuses amphetamine, a potentially dangerous combination of stimulants. Some recent deaths have been associated with herbal products that mimic Ecstasy, a mild hallucinogen. These products contain the stimulant ephedrine, which is also found in some (OTC) cold remedies.

*     *     *

The narcotic Vicodin was prescribed for Joan by an orthopedic surgeon whom she consulted several years ago. In general, she took no more than the prescribed amount, but she sometimes increased the dose for a day or two if the pain was unusually severe (on the first day of her menstrual period, for example).

Her prescription narcotic use may be interpreted in many ways: She may not actually has been abusing narcotics, since there was little evidence of specific negative consequences associated with their use. On the other hand, Joan made no real adjustments in her life to reduce the stress on her hip and consistently refused recommended surgery to correct her problem. Joan cited financial and emotional reasons for refusing surgery. She had no one to take care of her postsurgery, and she was afraid that she might be fired during her absence from work. Her refusal to go along with medical recommendations could be an example of poor self-care skills. Bear in mind, however, that since surgeons often recommend surgery, Joan's refusal may have been a red herring in terms of drug use, representing instead attitudes toward physicians in general and surgery in particular. In any case, although long-term use of narcotics is associated with physiological dependence, it does not tend to cause any significant medical problems. The problem with Vicodin, however, is that it contains acetaminophen, which in large quantities over time can cause serious liver problems.

Joan was not at that time currently using any other types of medication or preparation on a regular basis. She did take one multivitamin capsule and the herb echinacea for general immune system enhancement each day. She had shown some tendency in the past to alter dosages and duration of medical prescriptions, but she reported minimal consequences.

## Past Treatment History

Gathering information about past treatment history often leads to interesting but difficult-to-interpret findings. For instance, the fact that a client may have sought drug treatment two or more times in the past *could* indicate motivation and be a sign of eventual success. On the other hand, such a history could have more ominous implications for prognosis. It is important for the clinician gathering details about past treatment history to ask about treatment settings. The treatment modality should be identified (inpatient, residential, outpatient) because the clinician needs to investigate whether a particular person who remains sober for a year in a residential program is the type to relapse quickly in outpatient follow-up, or whether a person who has done quite well in self-help groups might relapse during the holidays, for instance. What type of program was it? How long did treatment last? Were there particular aspects of the treatment the client found helpful or did not like? This information assists the clinician in planning for the next phase of treatment matching. As an example of the importance of past treatment history and its relation to treatment matching, consider the 12-Step programs. Many people object to 12-Step programs for numerous reasons. Some find the spiritual/religious nature of this approach objectionable. Other individuals do not feel comfortable in a group setting; still others may find specifics unpalatable or unhelpful, such as the slogans or the pressure to attend a specific number of meetings each week. Of course, clients may object to some elements while finding others helpful. For example, the group sharing or being paired with a sponsor may help ease clients' sense of isolation.

The therapist needs to explore carefully the client's feelings and objections about past treatment attempts without automatically assuming that these objections represent resistance. If a client has used 12-Step groups in the past and is open to returning to one, the ability to voice objections might make the program more workable the next time. For clients whose negative opinions about some form of treatment, whether it be a 12-Step program or groups in general, are solid, it would be a mistake for a therapist to insist on their participation in an objectionable form of treatment. This discussion of past treatment is a crucial part of the assessment in that it not only supplies needed information to plan a more effective treatment method, but also the therapeutic relationship can be weakened or strengthened by the interaction between client and therapist. Respect for the client's perceptions is crucial to building a solid bond, and failure to secure the bond is a frequent cause of treatment dropout and failure.

Past treatment history should also include informal attempts by the client to seek help. Some people may try personal solutions such as reducing the substance intake or quitting on their own or with a group of friends. This method of enlisting the help of friends has often been successful for smokers. To further understand the client's perception of what was and was not helpful, such personal efforts should be explored. Once again, it is important to view attempts at controlling use as a positive stage of change and to resist labeling a person's efforts as denial of the need to become abstinent.

Information about past treatment can also be a way to assess clients' honesty, behavioral traits, intelligence level, psychological sophistication, and ability for introspection. Blaming a particular program for treatment failures may or may not be accurate, but externalizing blame as a *general* trait could indicate to the therapist that a client will have difficulty with any treatment that does not make use of his own opinions and efforts to change substance use patterns. It is important for the therapist to be aware of any such intense transference experiences, as these may be related to eventual success or failure.

Gathering information on past treatment clearly is not so simple as to have the patient fill out a form with places and dates. Again, the MAP is not only an information-gathering tool, but it is also a vehicle for the development of a working alliance with the client.

\* \* \*

Joan has gone to AA meetings several times during the previous 5 years. Each time, she quickly met another program member, and they would have a brief and intense affair, both relapsing in the process. When asked about this pattern, Joan readily acknowledged that it appeared to be a great avoidance strategy and wondered if she might be afraid of not using drugs or alcohol. Upon further questioning, Joan revealed that each time she tried to stop using, either in a 12-Step group or on her own, she became seriously depressed and suicidal within 3–4 weeks. The intensity of her feelings has always led to relapse.

Joan had never been in individual psychotherapy but has participated in couple counseling twice before. She found couple counseling painful, and still felt a lot of resentment about the counseling process and the therapists involved. Joan said the therapists always seemed to be more on her partner's side and that the relationships broke up as a result of the couple counseling. Still ambivalent about individual psychotherapy, Joan nonetheless felt a need to try to get her life together.

## Support System

Personal biases and the influence of provider cultures are most crucially evident in evaluating a client's *support system*. Psychology and psychotherapy traditionally use theories developed exclusively by Western-educated Caucasian professionals. These ideas assume the existence of universal developmental "tasks" and healthy adult personality traits and patterns. Individual autonomy and independence are not only valued, but also are often construed as the only possible outcome of healthy development. This emphasis on autonomy may, in fact, contribute to the increase in substance abuse that we have seen over the past 20 years by forcing children to abandon safe, nurturing relationships too early in a modern, complex life (Walant, 1995).

Our culture's emphasis on individual autonomy also colors our attitudes about support systems. Evaluating a support system is further complicated by the introduction of concepts such as "codependency" and "enabling" that are often rigidly applied to the people who constitute a client's support system. Such terms often cause one to characterize helpful, supportive efforts as pathological, and to assume that these behaviors promote or allow the other person's substance abuse to continue. Cultural patterns that value extensive interaction and behavioral support as well as the extended support systems of traditional and nontraditional families (gays and lesbians, for example) are too often criticized and excluded from the client's treatment.

At its best, a client's support system functions like a family and often consists of and/or resembles in some way the family of origin and its values, as well as the values of the larger culture. Knowing the number of people clients know they can count on is an important part of evaluating client needs during and after treatment. A client's sense of which relationships are most stressful, critical, or sabotaging of efforts to improve is equally important. Answers to questions about family members' substance use and their attitudes about the client's use are essential.

When evaluating the client's support system, the clinician should be cautious about using popular jargon such as "enabling" or "codependency." These once useful ideas have been misapplied so frequently that they can impede client understanding of problems or be used by the therapist primarily to express frustration or disapproval (see Gordon & Barrett, 1993). *Enabling* describes actions that foster the development and maintenance of addictive behaviors. Enabling behavior can take the form of not recognizing that an addiction problem exists, avoidance of dealing with it, protecting the other person from consequences of his or her behavior, controlling the user's behavior, or rescuing, by taking over that person's responsibilities. *Codependency* refers to unhealthy adjustments made by other people in relation to the user/abuser. A codependent person's attention shifts from his own needs to the demands and activities of the alcoholic or addict. While both terms describe important addiction dynamics, they are too often used unproductively. It is easy to see how some of these dynamics can hinder the acknowledgment of a substance abuse problem, but it is just as easy to see how some "rescuing" behaviors often save the family from greater harm. The example from Chapter 1 is relevant here. Maria, the wife who called her husband's boss when he had a hangover, provides a common example of the types of behavior described as pathological codependency. If Maria's behavior kept the husband working and bringing in a paycheck, who is to say that the family would be better served if he lost his job because she would not protect him from the consequences of his alcohol problem?

It is also a mistake to think of these concepts in purely psychological terms, when, in fact, they are culturally loaded. The expectation of significant behavioral support is higher in some cultures than in others. For many nonwhite and non-Western people, what might be called codependent behaviors are normal, expected aspects of interpersonal relationships. To suggest otherwise is detrimental to the therapeutic relationship.

While the treatment outcome literature affirms the importance of supportive family and network members, clients' "significant others" are frequently confused about what constitutes appropriate engagement and detachment. During assessment, the clinician should review previous efforts by friends and family to cope with the situation, aiming to fine-tune productive efforts and discourage actions that are not. At some point in treatment, the clinician might want to discuss the idea of *enabling* as a way to help family members assess their own behavior and to discourage inappropriate forms of support. Such discussion elicits more precise descriptions and helps to clarify appropriate behaviors for support system people.

Family and support members can assist a client's recovery process in important ways: facilitating access to and participation in a treatment program; removing substances from the home; attending self-help meetings with the client; offering comfort and encouragement during difficult periods; and, most importantly, supporting the client even during an episode of relapse. The treatment plan should also achieve the following:

- Identify the needs of family and support people for information and assistance.
- Identify maladaptive coping patterns and specify what is needed to address them.

- Validate and fine-tune constructive actions.
- Define supporters' participation in the work to follow.

Each client needs to create her "family" according to what feels right to *her*. Despite the current "New Age" obsessions with intimacy and deep emotional "sharing," individual differences will always exist in levels of communication, contact, and emotional closeness. Some people can be reserved, aloof, or self-contained without being pathological. On the other hand, whereas significant social isolation is generally not therapeutic for a client (often indicating depression or other pathology), some individuals cannot tolerate much interpersonal interaction without becoming stressed or overwhelmed. Such people are sometimes schizophrenic, have strong schizoid traits, or are survivors of childhood abuse.

While the client needs to construct her support "family" in her own way (be it same-sex couples, unmarried heterosexuals, extended family, or friendship networks), the clinician needs to be aware of individual and cultural differences about standards for independence and intimacy. Shame and secrecy, verbal disclosure and emotional expressiveness, the willingness to use treatment groups, and other issues may vary greatly among individuals and in different cultures. For example, the cross-generational changes that occur in immigrant groups often cause significant distress and conflict for families in which the younger generation is assimilating. These families are stressed by value shifts that can make it difficult for the clinician to determine treatment strategies and goals.

But the most important issue for the clinician to assess is whether the client has significant support available to her, and whether she can utilize it in times of distress. Again, any dynamics the therapist presumes are detrimental should be evaluated in light of varying cultural norms.

\*     \*     \*

Joan had no close friends or family where she lived or in her hometown. Significantly, it was Joan's problem in sustaining relationships that brought her into treatment. While her work history was stable, Joan made only superficial friends at work.

Also a lesbian, Joan spent much of her time within the lesbian subculture. Unlike a more typical lesbian pattern of developing some friendship prior to initiating sexual contact, Joan's style was to meet a new woman and become sexual immediately. This "instant intimacy" quickly became problematic for her. In clinical interviews, Joan was articulate and intelligent, and displayed an infectious sense of humor. Given these personality traits, it is surprising that she had no close friends. This fact obviously reflects the level of psychopathology that must have been present in Joan's interpersonal relations.

## Self-Efficacy

As stated earlier, a person's sense of power, control, and confidence is essential to self-esteem and to the ability to make significant, difficult changes. A person's level of self-efficacy is not, however, a static thing. Each person has a general, or global, sense of self-efficacy: how much he feels that things generally work out for him; how confident he is that he can pretty much count on himself to do well; how he feels other people react to him. Many subtle differences might appear, however, when you ask this same man to describe his confidence in other, more specific abilities: How confident is he that he could give a speech in front of a large audience? Would he be able to disagree with his boss, and so forth? While the details of such self-efficacy will certainly emerge throughout the course of treatment, and particularly when working on relapse prevention, it is helpful to get some sense of the person's feelings of self-confidence in different areas of his life early in the assessment process. Deficits in global self-efficacy are a serious concern when changing addictive behaviors and need to be addressed directly in psychodynamic psychotherapy in order for any stable change to occur. Specific areas of deficits may or may not be important; if so, they can often be dealt with by shorter-term cognitive and behavioral methods.

*       *       *

Joan showed extremely variable self-efficacy in all areas of her life. She felt very confident in her intellectual abilities and her ability to use her intelligence to advance professionally. Aware that she was attractive to other people, both physically and in terms of her personality, particularly her sense of humor, she was not shy about initiating contact with new people. She was, however, terrified of new environments (a fact that was later to result in her terminating therapy), and could not go to a new place without checking the route many times. She had missed career and social opportunities because of her tendency to indulge in this fear and not do the practice that she knew would help. In terms of her mental health, Joan felt very strongly that she could not live without using drugs or alcohol, that the depression and pain she felt whenever she tried to quit would overwhelm her, and that she would commit suicide. This opinion of herself as a weak, helpless person underlay and undermined other areas of her self-esteem and was a major barrier to treatment.

## Psychiatric Diagnosis

The presence of significant psychopathology that constitutes a *psychiatric diagnosis* complicates client assessment and treatment. Substance use may mimic a psychiatric disorder, exacerbate it, or reduce symptomatology, at least temporarily (Evans & Sullivan, 1990). Schizophrenic clients who use cocaine often exhibit fewer of the negative symptoms (anhedonia, cognitive decline, social withdrawal, etc.) that are characteristic of their disorder, even though they may have acute episodes of positive symptoms on a more frequent basis. Some people who depend on alcohol become depressed with long-term use, but in a certain subset of women, alcohol use appears to prevent or reduce depressive symptoms. Speculation is that alcohol interacts with both the estrogen and dopamine system in females in a way that improves mood. Anxiety may either be soothed or exacerbated by marijuana use. Stimulants often cause an acute depressive state even in otherwise healthy people, and can induce psychosis in vulnerable people. These substance effects vary among individuals, making assessment a daunting task, and even more so when dealing with clients who have been previously assessed with a dual diagnosis. The clinician must often make several "rule out" diagnoses during the assessment process until laboratory tests or time help clarify the symptom picture.

In order to understand accurately the interplay between psychiatric, substance induced, and characterological traits, the clinician must take a longitudinal view and be willing to listen to the client's perceptions of drug effects. One's professional knowledge of pharmacology is important as a guide, but it cannot be assumed to be the final statement of drug effects on an individual. We have all noticed persons who become funloving after a few drinks, as well as the ones who become morose. Individual differences have a potent, and sometimes contradictory, effect in combination with different substances and in different situations. Outcome expectancies heavily influence not only the type of drug used, but also the effects and pattern of use (Marlatt & Gordon, 1985).

Chapter 6 presents more information on dual diagnoses and a detailed case study of a patient with multiple diagnoses.

*       *       *

Joan exhibited significant symptoms that suggest character pathology. Though she had no current symptoms consistent with any Axis I diagnosis other than polysubstance abuse or dependence, it appears that she experienced significant depressive symptoms when not using substances. During both intake and later sessions, Joan described the following symptoms:

- Long-standing affective lability.
- Poor affect tolerance and modulation.
- Chaotic and demanding interpersonal relationships.
- Excessive fears of abandonment.
- Self-destructive behaviors (substance use).
- Feelings of emptiness.

This symptom cluster is consistent with a diagnosis of borderline personality disorder. It is possible, however, that some lability may be secondarily caused by the use of alcohol and cocaine. She also may have had either an independent affective disorder (major depression) or a substance-induced affective disorder; however, her rapid development of serious dysphoric symptoms upon abstinence from alcohol suggests that alcohol was acting to suppress, rather than increase, dysphoria. Thus, an independent affective disorder is more likely. As her psychiatric symptoms and drug use have coexisted for a long time, it is impossible to be completely certain of this diagnosis. Treatment needed to proceed with this provisional diagnosis, with further reassessment if and when drug-free periods were established.

The psychodynamically trained clinician will also notice the possibility of an anaclitic-like depression (Blatt, 1974). A history of significant early loss combined with a symptom picture of longing, clinging dependency, and the absence of guilt suggest a characterological depression (the next DSM may actually include such a diagnosis). This diagnostic picture suggests the importance of not only in-depth psychotherapy but also the use of psychiatric medications to support such a fragile patient. Therapeutic confrontation should be kept at a minimum with such a patient. Her psychosocial history, drug use, the suicide of her brother, and increasing social problems made her a serious suicide risk, particularly in the early stages of abstinence from alcohol.

## Clients' Stated Goal(s)

Some clients already have their goals in mind when they enter treatment. Others have given little thought to the options, while still others assume that total abstinence is the only legitimate or acceptable goal. Simple questions at the start of assessment, such as, "What would you like to change?" or "How do you see yourself being different after therapy?" can initiate a conversation about goals that may take many sessions to complete. The clinician should remember that such questions may be construed by the client as traps: He *knows* what the correct answer should be, so why is the therapist creating a subterfuge by asking (Mark & Faude, 1997)? Many others have already addressed the problem of goal setting in substance abuse treatment (Rotgers, 1998).

In behavioral terms, a well-formed treatment goal involves specific, observable behavioral changes that are achievable within the context of the client's life (Berg & Miller, 1992). Keep in mind that a client's goals may be immediate, short-term or long-term in their timing.

### Sample Client Goals

- Stop drinking within 2 months.
- Quit smoking crack today.
- Quit smoking pot this week, and quit cigarettes in 3 months.
- Only have two drinks per day and no pot starting now.
- Only snort speed, no more using needles.
- Quit drinking altogether for 3 months, then have only one drink per day.

It is clear from these examples that patient goals range from total, immediate abstinence to moderation and harm reduction while continuing active use. As the therapist works with the client, the goals should derive from the unique decisional balance worksheet, with the therapist guiding the process rather than offering opinions.

Other treatment goals may be more or less explicit between client and therapist. Changes in psychodynamic structure and functions such as affect modulation, impulse control, flexible defenses, and so forth, are indications of success and thus constitute important goals of treatment.

Clients may also have more or less clear ideas about the type of treatment and the setting desired. Some clients will be adamant either for or against hospitalization, going to 12-Step meetings, or other treatment choices. Others may have limited knowledge about the options available and will need to rely on the therapist for education and recommendations.

\*       \*       \*

Initially, Joan's goals were vague, based as much upon her assumptions about what would be acceptable to me as they were on her own wishes. She was clearly frightened to make any changes since her previous attempts to quit using drugs and alcohol had resulted in serious depression and suicidal feelings. She also had different concerns about the different drugs she was using.

Eventually (within 3 months), Joan stated a series of short-term goals that were interesting in that they reflected her measurement of how much change she wanted to undertake at one time:

- Quit shooting cocaine now.
- Reduce alcohol consumption to two drinks per day.
- Limit prescription Percodan to three pills per day.
- Snort cocaine only once per week for now.
- Stop smoking pot completely.

Joan was also adamant about not going into a hospital or residential program because she wanted to keep her job, an important source of self-esteem and income. She was reluctant to attend 12-Step meetings because of her past history of sexual involvement with other program members. Joan's hope was that individual therapy would be sufficient treatment.

## Therapist's Stated Goals

During assessment, the therapist forms hypotheses about the client's degree of addiction and a number of psychological variables. On the one hand, some therapists begin the process with predetermined ideas about what constitutes appropriate treatment goals. The old standard of waiting until a person is ready to quit, or refusing to see clients until they have already achieved some level of abstinence (24 hours to 1 month in some programs) is as widely applied as ever. On the other hand, some therapists may tend to underestimate the influence of substances on patients' psychological presentation and conduct treatment, believing that substance use is only a symptom of an underlying disorder and drug or alcohol use does not need to be addressed. In this context, another look at Joan's case helps to elucidate the process of identifying the *therapist's goals*.

\*      \*      \*

Joan was emotionally fragile and had a history of major psychiatric disturbance during sobriety. As her therapist, I would be wise to use a harm reduction strategy for early stages of treatment, knowing that this phase would probably last a year or more. In this particular case, Joan's stated goals might have been acceptable *so long as I communicated a professional concern that controlled use ultimately might not work for her.*

Treatment goals might include developing coping resources and other ego skills related to affect tolerance, self-care when in distress, and a solid therapeutic relationship that would be measured by Joan's consistent attendance, her willingness to call me when in distress, and some kind of statement by Joan that the therapy was helpful.

Joan needed a strong bond with me in order to address underlying issues and do further work on her significant relationship with drugs. Session frequency could have been increased to twice weekly when the therapeutic work shifted from ego building to an exploration of Joan's core issues. Bear in mind that hospitalization, medications, and other resources might have been an important part of the treatment plan at a later time.

## Developmental Grid

The developmental grid (Adelman & Bar-Hamburger, 1994) was developed as a teaching tool for psychiatrists in psychodynamic training. This grid is based on Khantzian's self-medication hypothesis, which asserts that there is an important relationship between the drug of choice, its pharmacological effects, and the core affective struggles in the individual with substance abuse problems.

This grid allows psychodynamically informed clinicians to utilize their skills to formulate "genetic" determinants, developmental sequences, deficits and compensatory mechanisms, and, ultimately, a coherent treatment plan. This more comprehensive treatment formulation has not been possible in other psychodynamic treatment orientations because other viewpoints focus selectively on only some of these components. Khantzian's model asserts that there are several characteristic psycho-pathological mechanisms at work in a person who develops a serious substance abuse problem:

- Defenses versus overwhelming anxiety.
- Other affects, such as rage, shame, and loneliness.
- Compensation for these overwhelming feelings.
- A "method of tempering" defenses.

The developmental grid, useful for other theoretical orientations as well, is presented in Figure 3.3 as a general format for thinking about history and treatment implications.

This grid makes it easy to assign specific historical events to their relative place in the psychological development of the individual. The clinician can then use different theoretical orientations to complete the analytical process inherent in the model. The assumption in the grid is that *significant developmental events* (Column 1) have a direct relationship to the development of *personality traits* (Column 2). This standard theoretical assumption in psychodynamically oriented psychotherapy has not been routinely assessed in chemical dependency treatment.

This model further asserts a definable *relationship between a*

| Significant developmental event | Personality traits shaped by this event | Relationship of trait to genesis of addictive disorder | Relationship of trait to treatment and recovery process |
|---|---|---|---|
|  |  |  |  |

FIGURE 3.3. The developmental grid.

*particular personality trait and the genesis of the addictive disorder* (Column 3). Chemical dependency theories do not focus on specific developmental factors and thus lack a "richness" that is important in treating individuals. Most importantly, however, is the next point of Khantzian's theory, which departs radically from both traditional chemical dependency and psychodynamic therapeutic approaches. Khantzian states that there is a specific *relationship between the personality trait that has genetic implications and the actual treatment/ recovery process* for substance abuse (Column 4).

Whereas few clinicians think of substance-abusing clients in this manner, it is a common conceptual process for other disorders. Clinicians assume treatment is characterized by emerging repetitive patterns that must surface and be reworked in order to produce lasting therapeutic benefit. Chemical dependency treatment can also use such individual discriminations instead of relying only on broad, group-based characteristics.

*        *        *

A wealth of information exists concerning significant developmental events that shaped Joan. Both of her parents were killed in a car accident when she was 5 years old, after which she was sent to an orphanage with her older brother. Joan lived there until she was 11 and suffered physical abuse from orphanage staff.

In utilizing the developmental grid, the focus here is on only one distinct event, the death of Joan's parents when she was 5. Thus, I would enter *Death of Parents* in Column 1. It could be hypothesized that several of Joan's personality traits were shaped by her parents' death. To assume abandonment fears, Oedipal anxieties, and other issues would all be appropriate. For this example, the focus on Joan's *Abandonment Fears* would be entered in Column 2.

These fears would certainly play an important part in the development of an addictive disorder in several ways. Joan's drug use might have been an *attempt to numb the painful affects of abandonment while temporarily suppressing anxieties about her interpersonal relationships*, noted in Column 3.

These issues related directly to the process of therapy, including Joan's *efforts to hide her strong dependency needs in order to avoid the abandonment feelings in her transference*, entered in Column 4, as were notes about how Joan's *vacillation between clinging or demanding interactions and distancing maneuvers might be expected*. Getting Joan to continue in therapy would be difficult, and her instincts to flee would need to be addressed early on in treatment.


## CONCLUSIONS


Assessment is clearly a detailed, often lengthy process in the treatment of substance use problems. The *sequence* of assessment information presented here is somewhat arbitrary; remember that in many cases, treatment also takes place concurrently with assessment. Once all the information is gathered it may be important for the therapist to decide if there are multiple diagnoses and, if so, which diagnosis is primary; this area is a source of much disagreement among treatment staff. Traditionally, the primary disorder is considered to be the one that presented earliest in the client's history. Joan's assessment clearly shows my bias toward assessing all disorders, without the need to label one as primary.

CHAPTER FOUR

---

# *Treatment Design:*
# *How to Think about a Case*

## THE FOUNDATIONS OF TREATMENT

It should be apparent that the assessment process detailed in the previous chapter is not intended to progress in a linear fashion or to result in a uniform treatment design applicable to all clients. Nor does the assessment process stand by itself as a discrete process. Much of the information can be obtained during the course of the therapy itself, and it often works best that way. An overly formalized approach to assessment (i.e., conducting an assessment before initiating treatment) does not allow enough flexibility to respond to the client's immediate needs. Nor does it accommodate client defenses against revealing sensitive, personal details to a stranger. Information may be obtained, but sometimes at the expense of the development of a trusting and cooperative therapeutic alliance. The principles of motivational interviewing stress the importance of developing a working relationship as the first step in any treatment process. *Harm reduction psychotherapy rests on the belief that the interactions within a relationship between the drug user and the clinician help create the environment within which change takes place.* Whether the relationship consists of a one-time meeting, ongoing case management, or an extended psychotherapy, it is essential to take the time to build mutual trust and cooperation.

This chapter prepares the reader to develop an individualized treatment plan for each patient by discussing (1) the foundations and process of harm reduction psychotherapy, and (2) several critical theoretical constructs that guide the treatment process.

## Developing Rapport

Every clinician has learned that developing rapport is the basic foundation of psychotherapy. Working with people who have drug or alcohol problems demands that the clinician take special care to counteract the negative stereotypes that lead the therapist to mistrust the patient and patients to shy away from the full truth regarding their problems. The primary attitude should be one of "Tell me what is bothering you," and, more importantly, "tell me how *you* see your problems." The pull to jump in with solutions or confrontations is great when a client is obviously ruining her life, but premature action on the therapist's part often ruptures rapport. Sometimes, doing nothing is the best therapeutic intervention.

## Modeling Curiosity

Because people with drug and alcohol problems come to treatment with excessive guilt, worry, and shame, they also tend to be self-critical, even self-hateful. Oftentimes, the exploration of their behaviors leads to increased self-loathing and dysphoria that can derail treatment at the earliest stages. The therapist needs to be prepared to model an attitude of curiosity about the complexities of people's experience and actively help them resist both self-hatred and any habit of minimizing the importance of their drug use.

## First Things First

While it may seem obvious, the first treatment decision to be made is often thrust upon us by some emergency. Suicidality, whether from depression or stimulant withdrawal, must be addressed with strong measures. Medical conditions, child abuse, or psychotic thinking also may require immediate intervention that has little to do with drug treatment. The therapist's rule of thumb, as in dealing with all patients who present for treatment, is to stabilize the most dangerous symptoms first, creating a safety net to catch the person before attempting any interventions that may cause psychological stress. Once the person is out of immediate danger, the therapeutic process can proceed.

Despite the often compelling nature of drug problems in the treatment setting, the therapeutic process requires attention to the client's immediate needs. A man with no money for food, even if it is because he spent it on drugs, is in crisis and should be given access to resources to feed himself before any other topic is broached. Similarly, a woman who is late for appointments because of child care problems needs help in removing this barrier to treatment. The fact that many of a person's difficulties may be caused directly or indirectly by drug or alcohol use is irrelevant at the beginning of treatment. The goal is to bring the person into the room and to be helpful in order to convince him or her that the therapist has something to offer. Exploration of the interaction between drug use and life problems is a delicate process that, for many patients, needs to be postponed until the relationship is secure.

## Identifying Healthy Ambivalence: The Decisional Balance

Contrary to clinicians' fondly held beliefs, clients work best when tension is maintained between what they like about using drugs and the negative consequences that they suffer as a result. The therapist needs to resist the urge to join in patients' simplification of their drug use and premature formulation of needed changes. A simple, "I can see you understand that alcohol is causing enormous problems for you, yet drinking has been a central part of your life for a long time. It must also be important to you somehow. I'd like to know more about that as well," will keep patients open to exploring the complexities that maintain their relationship to alcohol.

The person who comes to treatment as a result of coercion may have a different problem, one of denying the existence of any serious consequences of his drug use. It is a mistake for the therapist to take on the other side of the patient's ambivalence in the mistaken belief that he needs to *develop insight* or *confront his denial*. The therapist's task is the same with both types of clients: Help the person realize the complex positive *and* negative reasons for drug use by modeling curiosity and resisting premature conclusions.

## A Word about Language

Different provider cultures each develop language and terminology of their own. Since language tends to reflect unstated beliefs, it is a good target for scrutiny. Jargon or specialized vocabularies create subcultures that differentiate provider cultures from each other and from the lay public. Language is a potent vehicle for asserting one's independence and uniqueness. The words we use both reveal and create attitudes that we hold about our patients, reflecting individual opinions and cultural biases.

Mental health clinicians tend to use words such as "transference" (to refer to the feelings and thoughts that our patients may have about us) and "resistance" (patients' reluctance to take what we say as true). These terms create a parallel relationship of which clients are generally not aware and in which they, therefore, are not active participants.

Just as mental health clinicians have culture-specific language, so do clients. This is especially true of drug users, who often belong to a particular subculture based partly on their drug of choice. Words such as *junkie, speed freak, doper,* or *tweaker* have particular meaning and are often terms of solidarity and mutual understanding, if not endearment. Just as gays and lesbians sometimes adopt the pejorative terms of society as words of pride, so do drug users. But just because a lesbian calls herself a "dyke" or a gay man refers to himself as a "faggot" does not mean that those terms are condoned or accepted when they come from outside the particular subgroup. There are numerous other examples of racial-, gender-, and culture-based words being used within a subculture in one context and simultaneously seen as pejorative when used by someone outside of the group. The fact that such terms are often reclaimed by a minority group points to the original hostile and demeaning attitudes that created them and opens a window of understanding into the self-hatred that so often haunts people who live within minority communities. A similar situation exists with drug users, who have been subjected to society's hostility and misunderstanding. They, too, may have adopted certain words that, reflecting the attitudes of others, contribute to the self-hatred and self-loathing that may underlie bravado.

The 12-Step self-help tradition has developed a language wherein certain words have been appropriated and idiosyncratically redefined by this culture and then erroneously considered definitive and absolute. People who attend 12-Step groups routinely refer to themselves as *addicts* and *alcoholics* in their introductions during meetings. Members of 12-Step groups also refer to themselves as being *in recovery* from drugs and alcohol. This term implies that one can never fully recover from an addiction and is in a process of lifelong recovery that requires vigilance and persistent self-scrutiny. The term also implies that the person is "working the program," that is, actively working through the 12 Steps as identified in what is called *The Big Book* (Alcoholics Anonymous, 1939/1976). Identifying oneself as being *in recovery* sends an in-group message that gains one instant recognition and acceptance from other people who are in 12-Step programs and sets them apart from others who at one time used drugs and no longer do. People *in recovery* are received with a special consideration and instantly feel the support offered by the community.

While members of 12-Step groups have adopted the term "in recovery," other people who are struggling with addictions have no terms to identify themselves and no group identity to offer them support and encouragement. These people represent the majority of persons with addictive problems but are not acknowledged by the 12-Step community as fellows in recovery, and are often considered suspect by clinicians who cannot quite believe that they have really overcome their addiction. In fact, research indicates that many people do change and/or resolve their addictions without any help from others (Sobell, Cunningham, & Sobell, 1996; Peele, 1991). There is nothing inherently wrong with creating a culture-specific language. I am simply pointing out the power of language to form group cohesion or, conversely, to alienate and isolate outsiders.

A similar situation exists regarding the term "in treatment," which generally refers to a person who is participating in an abstinence-based program. Even though 12-Step groups are considered to be self-help organizations and not treatment, the fact that 97% of all substance abuse programs in the United States use 12-

Step practices and groups as the primary vehicle for treatment means that there is a significant alliance between 12-Step groups and drug treatment. Judges often require that a person convicted of a drug-related offense be "in treatment" as a condition of probation. Attendance at 12-Step meetings often satisfies this requirement. It is still common for psychotherapists to require that a person be "in drug treatment" prior to being accepted into therapy. The message is clear: People with drug or alcohol problems can only work on their problems in the context of abstinence and 12-Step groups. Other components of treatment, such as skills training, relapse prevention, or family sessions, occur within the framework of 12-Step participation. Psychotherapy is not considered to be a legitimate treatment for such problems.

This use of the phrase "in treatment" has the same effect as the phrase "in recovery." It creates a hierarchy that separates the good clients from the not so good ones, the motivated from the unmotivated, the successes from the failures. The sense of pride and power gained by one's efforts at self-help is not offered to those outside the group.

Even though harm reduction therapy is relatively new in the United States, the phrase has already been defined. This process of definition is unique in that it has taken place because of an odd congruence of workers in the harm reduction movement and chemical dependency specialists, who generally have little upon which to agree. Erroneously, "harm reduction" is taken to mean *non*abstinent. Someone practicing "harm reduction" supposedly is against abstinence-oriented treatment, interested only in efforts to reduce the harm associated with *continued* drug use. This restriction of the term is unfortunate, as it serves to alienate groups of people, all of whom are interested in finding effective ways of treating substance use problems.

In conclusion, the restrictive use of language, or the pressure to be politically correct regarding language, can divert attention from good works and good people who do not use the words we feel are respectful. Often, the best a clinician can do is engage in a dialogue with each person and develop sufficient flexibility and respect for the ideas of the other that a bridge can be built, a compromise formulated, that allows the important work of psychotherapy to begin.

# TREATMENT MATCHING

Treatment matching is a relatively new concept in the chemical dependency field. Research has shown that not everyone benefits from the same type or intensity of treatment. Despite popular belief, there is little evidence that 12-Step programs are any more effective than other forms of treatment (Bower, 1997; McLellan et al., 1997; and Project MATCH Research Group, 1997), at least in the in the treatment of alcoholism. The Project MATCH study concludes that, other than patients with severe psychiatric symptoms, one need not take into account client characteristics when matching patients to treatment modalities. This shows the willingness of researchers to ignore certain problems. The majority of patients do *not* succeed in maintaining abstinence with *any* of the offered treatments (about one in four maintained abstinence throughout the 1-year study). Researchers are saying that *all* types of drug treatment work, when it is more accurate to say that currently designed alcohol and drug treatments work for only a minority of patients, and we do not know what might work for the majority who do not stay in treatment.

Studies suggest that there may be patient and therapist characteristics that influence both acceptability of treatment and outcome. Yet, as of now, we have little to guide our clinical decision making. The following are some guidelines, however, that will assist the clinician in treatment planning.

## Provide a Menu

Choice is an important part of treatment. An expanding body of research indicates that the more options given to a patient, the better the treatment outcome. Choice empowers clients to be active and involved in their treatment and earn the respect of their therapist. In psychotherapy, it is assumed that the patient exercises a great deal of choice in treatment. Different clinicians offer a wide variety of intervention types (group therapy, body work, individual therapy, etc.) in a wide variety of settings (inpatient, day treatment, outpatient, etc.). Yet there are very few choices offered to people in chemical dependency treatment. This results not entirely from a lack of alternative approaches, but rather from a lack of knowledge or interest in pursuing different treatments. Choice is also often restricted by insurance reimbursement, employer rules, and the judicial system. (Rulings are pending in several cases charging that involuntary sentencing to 12-Step programs violates the person's right to freedom of religion.) Within these constraints, however, it is important to develop as specific a plan as possible with each individual.

The options should include alternatives and specialized planning in four areas: (1) treatment goals and hierarchy of needs; (2) level and intensity of intervention; (3) cultural competency; and (4) the specific types of interventions used.

## Treatment Goals

Clinician opinions vary widely on the importance and process of developing therapeutic goals, some preferring to think in development terms such as affect tolerance, ability to manage frustration, and so on. Others are more behavioral in their approach and use relatively measurable indices of success in treatment, such as a decrease in the number of panic attacks or an increase in social activities. Drug and alcohol problems lend themselves to behavioral-type treatment goals, but the relapse rate is still unacceptably high. While behavioral change is almost always going to be a part of harm reduction psychotherapy, the emphasis in the treatment may not always be on the drug use itself. The unique patterns of use, the relationship between clients and their drugs, and the risks and benefits of change are important aspect of treatment.

An integrated approach to treatment goals should take into account many factors. Rotgers (1998) summarizes the most recent available studies regarding choice of goals in chemical dependency work. He states that, despite the guidance provided by the research, clinical decisions are too often made on the basis of "philosophical considerations and anecdotal clinical lore rather than on empirical evidence supporting these practices" (p. 65). He cites a study concluding that when treatment goals are imposed upon a client in alcohol treatment, the outcome is negatively affected. This is true whether the imposed goal is abstinence *or* moderation (Sanchez-Craig & Lei, 1986).

Clinicians often assume that offering a choice (e.g., of goals regarding drinking) will allow a person to decide upon a harmful course of action, but that does not seem to be the case. Given a combination of unbiased information and empathic counseling, most clients will choose a goal that is appropriate to their level of difficulty with alcohol consumption, a goal that the clinician might have chosen for them (Ojehagen & Berglund, 1989; Pachman, Foy, & VanErd, 1978). These studies also show that between 50% and 84% of all clients entering treatment chose abstinence from alcohol. These studies can help to ease our fears that, given free choice, clients will always decide to continue drinking. We are not in danger of "enabling" a patient to continue alcohol abuse. Unfortunately, no studies of this type have been done with other drugs. My own clinical experience supports the research on alcohol: The majority of patients decide that abstinence (at least from their "drug of choice") is the most prudent course.

It is important to remember that treatment goals can consist of both short- and long-term options. In fact, it is often quite easy to convince patients to quit using a drug temporarily if they realize they can change their mind in the future, or if they wish to try moderation as a long-term goal. This combination of short-term and long-term goals is an important part of the treatment. For example, a person who is physiologically dependent on a substance finds it very difficult to moderate his use as a first step. The effects of tolerance and withdrawal make it unlikely that he will be successful in his efforts to cut down. A frank explanation of this physiological fact, along with an openness to alternative long-term goals other than complete abstinence, will often allow a client to consider short-term abstinence. In other cases, when a person is not physiologically dependent, she may be willing to try other harm reduction methods, such as "drug-free days" to reduce the most serious problems she is experiencing. Miller and Page (1991) describes three "warm turkey" alternatives to abstinence: tapering, trial moderation, and sobriety sampling. Rather than inadvertently encouraging future use, such approaches offer the client an experience of being drug free, or at least less intoxicated, as an option, and within the supportive hold of a therapeutic relationship.

## Building a Needs Hierarchy

A thorough assessment uncovers many different patient needs. In psychotherapy, the delineation of therapeutic "needs" is not often offered to the patient, and in chemical dependency treatment, the needs of clients are usually not considered beyond their "need" to quit using drugs and alcohol. In fact, patients bring with them many wishes and needs that must be addressed in order to make an empathic connection and ensure treatment retention. Treatment programs inadvertently create barriers for many people, barriers resulting from inadequate funding and staffing, as well as from ill-conceived "tests" of a client's motivation. Limited hours, locations removed from public transportation or in unsafe neighborhoods, lack of child care and transportation money, staffing patterns that do not reflect the racial or gender mix of clients, and so forth, are all real barriers to treatment.

One of the most important parts of treatment planning is the mutual development of a needs hierarchy, a statement of what the *patient* considers most immediate and crucial to the resolution of other problems. The clinician has input into this hierarchy by virtue of experience and information, even though it should be up to the client to make the final determination of what needs to be addressed first. For example, a young single mother who is using speed has many obvious problems that need to be addressed. A needs hierarchy developed by a traditionally trained counselor might look like the following:

> Stop using speed and all other drugs.
> Attend 12-Step meetings (often, the frequency of attendance is specified).
> Attend a drug treatment day program that will do urine testing to ensure abstinence.
> Attend stress reduction and parenting classes.
> Get a high school equivalency diploma.
> Get a job.

It is possible, of course, that the client will agree that this is the best plan for her. It is likely, however, that many young women in this position would come up with a slightly different needs hierarchy that might more closely resemble the following, taken from an actual case in which the client was able to articulate her needs clearly from the beginning:

> Get child care so I can reduce stress and "take care of business" (shopping, laundry).
> Have the counselor sign for disability or welfare benefits so that I can pay my rent tomorrow.

Keep my ex-boyfriend from coming around offering me drugs.
Figure out a budget so I won't have to steal to buy drugs or
   food.
Quit using speed every day.
Eventually get a job to take care of me and my kid.

We clinicians often think that we know the steps necessary for a
person to achieve a specific goal, and we find it hard to help a person
take a different route. Adopting such a supportive and actively helping stance, however, often reveals important surprises: People manage to decrease harm in their lives and arrive at healthier solutions
from many different directions. We must examine the reaches and
limits of our expertise when it comes to managing another person's
daily life. The goal in treatment is for the client—with the therapist—
to develop a needs hierarchy that is largely based on the client's perceptions of her tasks and her resources to accomplish her goals. The
therapist's role is to supply information and expertise that can help
the client determine her priorities.

## Level and Intensity of Intervention

Decisions about the best treatment setting or frequency are based as
much upon financial and lifestyle constraints as on considerations of
the efficacy of different treatments. Ideally, a patient would be referred to an inpatient program if detoxification is necessary or if abstinence cannot be achieved independently. However, limited insurance coverage or an inability to keep a job through such an absence
may necessitate the use of outpatient facilities. Child care responsibilities are a common source of difficulty for women, and there are few
residential or inpatient options available to them. On the other hand,
there is no evidence to support the notion that inpatient treatment is
more effective than outpatient treatment in the long run and for most
patients (Miller & Hester, 1986). Length of treatment is the only
consistent measure that predicts a positive outcome. With that in
mind, the initial location of the treatment program is of less importance than was once believed. Many think that inpatient treatment, if
not followed by intense outpatient work, actually undermines people's ability to make changes in their own world. Residential treatment or intensive day treatment programs are useful for people who

have severe problems and/or lack the social support or the emotional strength to establish sobriety outside of a controlled setting. However, since financial, job, or family responsibilities may make these options untenable for many people, it is important not to interpret clients' refusal to accept such a referral as resistance to treatment.

The use of group formats for chemical dependency treatment has been the standard for so long that it has almost become a fixed rule. While support from people with similar problems is often extremely valuable, many people do not work well in group formats and do not experience the support that they are told is there. A person expressing reluctance to undertake group treatment should not be required to undergo such treatment. Resistance to group work should not be construed as a sign of denial or lack of motivation. Rather, if the therapist has some reason to think that group would benefit a client, it is appropriate at some point to explore the person's reluctance and offer the opportunity to experiment with this type of therapy.

Given these constraints, there are no easy rules for how often persons should be seen or how structured a program they need. Patient preference, once the therapist has provided information about options, should be the rule for treatment selection. Unfortunately, as some of the following cases will show, even when it *is* necessary to have inpatient or intensive outpatient interventions, the fact that most existing programs are limited to abstinence-only approaches will prevent many patients from accepting a referral. In these cases, the individual therapist is left to provide as much treatment, support, and structure as possible.

### Culturally Specific Treatments

Clinicians are becoming increasingly aware of the impact of cultural differences on treatment. For the past 10 years, the terms "cultural sensitivity" and, more recently, "cultural competence" have been used to highlight the importance of culture in the conceptualization and implementation of services. The psychodynamic differences among cultures are significant. For example, the view of the self can be quite different depending on the culture. In Western cultures, it is assumed that as children grow, they develop an awareness of the distinction between their minds and bodies. This mind–body split is considered to be psychologically healthy. Those with more fluid boundaries in this regard are often said to be psychosomatic; in other words, they transfer emotional experience and conflicts to body systems and develop syndromes such as gastrointestinal complaints, headaches, and so forth.

Many cultures, however, do not split the self into mind and body but view the person as more integrated, with emotional/mental experience often felt or expressed by the body. This is but one of many cultural differences that needs to be understood in order to set aside our standard theoretical models and attempt to evaluate and treat clients using the values and standards of their culture.

Even more than understanding the patterns and beliefs of different groups of people, we must include members of different groups in the planning and delivery of services in order to reflect the subtle flavors of each group. For example, the level of acculturation of each person is an important variable. A first generation Asian American is likely to retain more obvious characteristics of her culture of origin than is a fourth-generation Asian American. These two groups may have little in common other than names and physical characteristics. Language, religion, beliefs, and patterns of relating, among other things, are likely to be very different.

We have become increasingly aware of differences related to sexual orientation. Gay men and lesbians form the largest group of sexual minorities, as they are present in large numbers in most communities. Other sexual minorities, such as transgender and transvestites, when mature, often migrate to larger cities where they can better find a community. Research indicates that being a member of a sexual minority is associated with an increased risk of substance abuse, partly because of the stress of discrimination, and partly because of the centrality of nightclubs and bars in gay community life.

It is also important to consider differences in gender as a cultural difference. The issues involved may be more apparent in certain groups (Muslim, Afrotribal, etc.), but even the differences between men and women's psychology in the United States are significant. Most research in chemical dependency has been conducted on men, as has almost all of the research in pharmacology. How the results apply to women is not known, but clinical experience points to significant differences in terms of drug of choice, patterns of use, physiological consequences, concurrent sociolegal problems, parenting styles, and psychiatric disorders. It is extremely important to consider the differential needs of female clients in order to increase attraction and retention in treatment.

Many clinicians are working in the area of culturally competent treatment modalities for people with alcohol and drug problems (Weibel-Orlando, 1987). A recent issue of the *American Journal on Addictions* (1996) devoted an entire section to the interaction of alcohol and ethnicity. As more practitioners focus on these group issues, the treatments we develop will have more appeal and perhaps more success with many more people.

## Specific Therapeutic Strategies

Harm reduction psychotherapy allows creativity in the design of treatment strategies. One basic approach is to pair interventions with the client's current stage of change. The following is a set of suggestion about cognitive interventions at different stages of change. This area is just now being developed and used to design treatment programs, as well as individual treatment (see Prochaska, Norcross, & DiClemente, 1994, Little, 1999).

1. *Precontemplation.* Educate about drug effects; develop discrepancy between drug use and person's other goals and values; do not avoid discussion of drugs and alcohol; do not make suggestions or push the person into action.

2. *Contemplation.* Explore ambivalence; do not take sides; develop the decisional balance. This is the most important of all the stages of change because it gives the fullest explanation of drug, set, and setting and allows the client to explore fully the complexities of the drug experience.

3. *Preparation.* Change becomes a priority; make realistic plans toward change; clinician says, "Yes, but," and "What if this doesn't work?"

4. *Action.* "Right-sized steps" (Little, 1999); that is, identify smaller parts of the larger behavioral change wanted; explore "How is this working?"; plan for high-risk situations.

5. *Maintenance.* Choose a support system that is personally and culturally relevant; explore "How is this working?"; focus in psychotherapy on core issues and unresolved developmental problems.

6. *Relapse.* View as a learning opportunity; "What didn't work?"; back to the drawing board.

7. *Termination.* A natural end to the focus on drugs or alcohol;

review progress; continue to work on psychological issues as needed; move fully into the world without worry of relapse.

This type of strategy ensures that the work keeps pace with the developing therapeutic relationship. Some clients might seem to allow disruption in the relationship, but lack of progress indicates that the therapist has moved too quickly. Other clients are quick to resist interventions that are not sensitive to their current stage of change.

Other strategies can follow from one's own theoretical orientation. It is important to remember, however, that techniques such as interpretation and confrontation, or processes such as the exploration of transference, usually have to wait until the relationship is well established. One can safely use these techniques, then, to help the client negotiate any of the stages of change. The clinical examples that follow in the next chapters detail these general guidelines.

## ESSENTIAL CONCEPTS IN TREATMENT

The topics that follow have all been discussed at length by other authors and are summarized and restated here as a guide to clinical thinking. When faced with a patient suffering from an alcohol or drug problem, it is not enough to conduct an assessment, not even the thorough assessment outlined in Chapter 3. In order to design treatment, it is necessary to build a working model of the complex interactions of biopsychosocial forces in each individual's life. Important also are the psychodynamic and cognitive concepts that bridge the gap between our understanding of other types of disorders and the addictive process. The following sections on trust, attachment, affect, coping skills, and neurobiology introduce the clinician to a rich body of research and theory that can be brought to bear on actual treatment strategies with particular patients.

### Trust

Mental health clinicians are underrepresented among chemical dependency workers. Our training has focused on psychological dynamics and the cognitive and behavioral sequelae of such internal forces. Whether trained primarily in psychodynamic theory and technique, systems theory, or cognitive models, we assume that people are willing to adopt the role of client, or patient, looking to us with some amount of trust and hope that we will understand and help them.

The person with alcohol or drug problems often comes to treatment with very different attitudes and expectations. Aware of the negative stereotypes and biases that are prevalent in our culture, these clients rightly assume that we therapists may hold such negative views of them as well. And since the predominant treatment for drug disorders is one based on the assumption that addicts deny or minimize their drug problems, the initial encounter between therapist and client can be fraught with unspoken dangers. Mark and Faude (1997), referring to their work with cocaine addicts, have described several "ready-made transferences and countertransferences" (p. 213) based on the realities of the interaction of societal values, client worries, and therapist suspicions. Central to their theme is the problem of intersecting expectations: The client expects to be controlled and does not want to be, and the therapist expects the client to want to be helped, to be willing to be controlled in some subtle way. When we view an addict as being a problem, or not motivated, or in denial, we are often speaking of this conflict of expectations.

Societal values enter into the treatment setting in sometimes subtle, often blatant ways. Each participant, patient and therapist, watches the other for signs that indicate trustworthiness. Most people's opinions about the trustworthiness of so-called addicts are gleaned from television programs, from the press, sometimes from their own experiences. Stereotyped images of drug addicts as thieves, even stealing their families and closest friends, create fear in the therapist, who wonders whether the vase in the waiting room is safe, or whether he left his wallet in a jacket in the hall closet. Patients have their own fears about trust. "Is the therapist afraid of me? Is he worried that I'll steal from him? Can I tell him that I do steal from people sometimes?"

Therapists also fear that drug-using patients will routinely lie about the amount and frequency of their drug use or attempt to hide negative consequences. On their part, patients may indeed be watching for signs of approval or disapproval, making decisions about how much they should admit, and wondering at what point the therapist will become alarmed and confrontational. "Is it okay to drink four beers? What if I say I drink eight?" These concerns are often silent partners in the therapy room, creating distance and mistrust as they remain unspoken.

Therapists often forget that people's level of truthfulness varies depending on any number of contingencies, including how the other person might treat them if what they disclose is illegal. In contrast to what they have learned in general psychotherapy training, clinicians who have read or been taught anything about drug problems are cautioned about the tendency of patients to lie, minimize, and so forth, not only about their drug use, but also about other aspects of their lives. Conducting treatment with this bias results in mutual mistrust and the inevitable victimization of patients by therapists who question their every statement.

Given that some people do misrepresent or lie directly about their actions and motivations, how do therapists approach patients who perhaps have compelling reasons to lie to themselves and to others? After all, lying is a very protective device, as known by all of us who lied as children to avoid getting into trouble with parents, teachers, and friends. Two techniques are helpful at the beginning of treatment. First, it is important for the clinician to state clearly that the patient has a right to decide how to conduct his life, and that her job is to help him make his own decisions in that regard. While this statement alone will not reassure a person accustomed to having his drug use misrepresented, it forms the basis for all other therapeutic interventions and will be tested for inconsistencies by the patient. This testing process involves the patient's ongoing scrutiny of the therapist's overt behavior and attitudes. Increasing honesty on the part of the patient will follow as he observes the therapist's consistency and respect. The patient might, for example, increase his drug use temporarily and check the therapist's response. It is also useful for the therapist to ask how comfortable the patient is talking about details of his drug use. If the patient is hesitant or appears suspicious, the therapist might ask whether he has concerns about her reactions, and validate the social basis for these concerns.

The essential therapeutic task with regard to trusting patients with drug or alcohol problems is to create an atmosphere wherein the patient feels understood rather than judged. A silent, noncommittal (neutral) attitude usually will not be sufficient to accomplish this task. The therapist, understanding both the societal and personal basis for the patient's qualms about honesty, as well as the possibility of countertransference interference, must actively engage the patient in a discussion of these potential problems.

## Attachment

People with drug or alcohol problems develop relationships that are often influenced by societal values and negative experiences with helpers. In the previous section, I discussed the relationship between patient and therapist and how trust needs to be developed. *Drug users also develop complex relationships with the drugs that they use.* Of all of the psychological theories that exist, attachment theory, which is based on biopsychosocial research, offers the best way to understand the relationship that develops between users and their drugs. Problems of attachment in the interpersonal sphere often lead to an attachment to things not human. The interaction between these two spheres creates the unique set of relationships that characterizes the life of someone who has a drug problem.

Attachment theory rests on both observation and research, concluding that all humans are inherently motivated to maintain proximity to an important nurturing figure. This motivation results in a complex array of what Bowlby (1982, 1988) and Ainsworth (1982) call "attachment behaviors." These researchers have observed three distinct types of attachment styles in children, only one of which is considered normal and healthy. In general, a child who is well cared for, both physically and emotionally, develops a sense of well-being, of having a "secure base" from which to explore the world. This is termed *secure* attachment. Other children, because of neglect or trauma, do not develop a sense of security and show one of two insecure styles of attachment: *ambivalent* (anxious) or *avoidant* (detached). The securely attached child explores her environment, takes risks, and rushes to "home base" (the caretaker) when she is scared or needs comfort. The ambivalently attached child is often clinging and demanding, but at other times, she is hesitant to go to the caretaker. Avoidant children refuse contact with the caretaker and may appear aloof and independent rather than insecure. The style of attachment developed in childhood is solidified by about the age of 6, meaning that new attachments tend to be developed along the same lines, for better or worse, as the original attachments in infancy and young childhood. It takes concentrated intervention to change this basic blueprint for interpersonal relationships.

Consistent with the philosophy that underlies harm reduction psychotherapy, I believe that having an attachment to drugs or alcohol is not necessarily pathological. Such relationships, just like attachments to people, run the gamut from healthy and productive to destructive, from securely attached to anxious or avoidant. Therapists have a tendency to suspect that any regular use of drugs or alcohol indicates an unhealthy process, as if people were supposed to live their lives without the pleasurable or pain-relieving properties of all psychoactive substances. People who end each work day with a glass or two of wine generally do not arouse concern. If they indicate that to go without would be difficult for them, they are often categorized as having an alcohol problem, as are those who drink to the point of intoxication, or those whose drinking causes secondary life problems. (In a similar vein, some therapists would see dependency on a person as a possible indication of psychopathology. *Needing* another person for one's sense of stability and pleasure in life has become almost as suspect as needing a drink).

Walant (1995) offers a sophisticated and troubling view of this aspect of Western culture:

> Our society's long-standing denial and devaluation of merger phenomenon throughout the life cycle have actually increased the likelihood of personality disorders and addiction, precisely because autonomy and independence have been encouraged *at the expense of* attachment needs. . . . Beneath the veneer of self-reliance lies the core of powerlessness, alienation, and detachment. (p. 2)

Walant asserts that this devaluation of attachment needs is a primary cause of addiction in our culture and stands in stark contrast to most non-Western cultures. In the United States, children are encouraged to develop autonomy, and adults are expected to be independent. This independence seems to conflict with our "family values." We are expected at once to stand on our own two feet and to forge lasting bonds with others.

Walant uses terms such as "empathic attunement" and "merger experiences" to communicate the basic need for attachment experiences throughout the life cycle. Both of these terms refer to typical experiences between an infant and mother: The mother who knows her baby's different types of distress cries is exhibiting empathic attunement; holding and mutual gazing are examples of merger experiences between members of this dyad. Walant sees society's parenting practices as a form of "normative abuse . . . that occurs when the attachment needs of the child are sacrificed for the cultural norms of separation and individuation" (p. 8). This insistence on autonomy in a young child causes such distress to the child, she believes, that it represents a serious break in empathy. Such empathic breaks are the ultimate cause of an emotional detachment that paves the way for addiction.

According to attachment theory, detachment is the final response of the child to abandonment (Bowlby, 1988). Such children may appear self-assured and independent but often have an underlying anxious or avoidant style of attachment that drug addiction mimics. The patterns of intense drug craving (ambivalent attachment to the drug) and the concurrent lack of self-care (avoidant attachment to the self) can be seen as representations of these two styles of attachment. The user's intense efforts either to maintain proximity to the drug or to avoid it completely show the typical all-or-none relationship that people can develop with drugs. Unfortunately, it is precisely this all-or-none attitude that lies at the core of traditional drug treatment.

The works of Bowlby and Walant are a rich source of therapeutic ideas and intervention strategies for the treatment of addictions. While drug use patterns, like relationship patterns, exist on a continuum from healthy to pathological, it is clear that some patterns are an expression of unmet needs from an earlier development period. Those whose relationship with drugs results in serious harm have most likely sought out drugs as a substitute for intimate relationships, a search caused by early distress at the hands of caretakers. As adults, an inability to form lasting intimate relationships is an indication of such a developmental trauma. Indeed, persons can be unaware that they even have a strong emotional attachment to a person or a drug until they are threatened with abandonment or, in the case of drugs, withdrawal (Gorman, 1994, 1998). The retreat from human interaction leaves the person without a solid core of identity, power, and hopefulness.

In developing their own therapeutic approach, clinicians would be wise to investigate the rich literature regarding these theoretical constructs (e.g., Krystal & Raskin, 1970; Levin, 1991; Wurmser, 1978).

One of the most intriguing and difficult dilemmas is that the use of drugs, while adaptive in many ways in a person's life, may create serious impediments in psychotherapy. Since the therapeutic process is inextricably linked to an intimate relationship, the patient's attachment to people as well as to drugs is of concern. If drugs are primary attachment objects, therapists must proceed with caution, taking care to not strip the person of essential adaptive and defensive functions without offering effective substitutes. We, as therapists, offer ourselves as a substitute attachment, often without acknowledging the real limitations of that relationship: We are not readily available, nor are our efforts routinely successful. At the same time, what we offer patients is, we hope, an attachment experience that will build inner strength and the ability to relate more intimately to people.

This dominant position of drugs in the addict's psyche is often the identified reason that most authors and clinicians insist on abstinence as a condition, or primary goal, of treatment. They see any use of drugs as detrimental to the development of a therapeutic relationship and, ultimately, a healthy psyche. Harm reduction psychotherapy views drug use as a part of the person's internal makeup. Just as human relationships can be transformed by the therapeutic process, so can a patient's relationship to drugs or alcohol. Persons may choose to end or to alter significant relationships in their lives. Their relationship to drugs or alcohol is an example of a complex interaction of relationships and, just as in couple or family therapy, should be treated with respect and caution when therapeutic interventions are considered. It is also important to remember that attachments to drugs, as attachments to people or other activities, reside on a continuum from healthy to pathological. A person may become attached to alcohol or a drug as part of the normal development of a variety of sustaining relationships in his or her life.

## Personality Traits

Questions of etiologically significant experiences have plagued clinicians in all areas of psychopathology. The field of chemical dependency has not escaped this search for causality. Unfortunately, however, research has not supported any of the psychological models that have been proposed regarding the addictive personality (Miller, 1976; Skinner & Allen, 1983). People with addictive disorders are no more passive, oral, or characterologically disturbed than persons without drug problems. Nor do addicts use the defenses of denial and rationalization more than other clinical or nonclinical populations. The failure of research to confirm any of our fondest theories regarding vulnerability or personality traits has left us searching for other ways to pinpoint the obvious differences between people who develop serious drug disorders and those who do not. The "War on Drugs" points to exposure to drugs as the primary demon, but this does not seem to be an adequate explanation either. Most people who have access to alcohol and drugs do not use or abuse them. Nor are socioeconomic status, gender, or mental illness foolproof predictors, despite the increased vulnerability that these factors impose on a person.

Once a person has started to use a drug or alcohol, the impact of drug-specific pharmacology and brain reward mechanisms on drug-seeking behavior is apparent. However, other factors are at least as important in the *initiation* of drug use and the return to active use after a period of abstinence. The high rates of relapse cannot be accounted for solely by drug effects, not even by the newer theories regarding "delayed withdrawal syndromes." There are several empirical animal models that may account for drug seeking in the absence of an established physical dependency (Gardner, 1997). Prior experience and the setting in which drugs are used, play a large part in consumption patterns in animals. Apparently, stress-free drug-seeking behavior is not unique to humans. Stress, however, increases the pathological use of drugs, and continuous drug use can be assumed to have some psychodynamic and cognitive–affective origins.

The problem with assuming that personality traits are predictors of addiction can be solved by viewing these traits from a correlational rather than a causal level. Instead of seeking to prove that a certain trait is the *cause* of addiction, one might better describe traits that appear *with* addictive problems. One can then view personality traits as the conceptual bridge between a person's internal world and the external manifestations of it—his behaviors. For example, one person who uses marijuana often experiences the world (internally) as overwhelming. He then smokes pot (the behavior) and experiences a softening of the harshness of this vision. Clinicians may see this habitual behavior as an indication of an avoidant personality trait that *causes* the drug use, but it is just as likely that he has made a serendipitous discovery that is reinforced by the success in reducing his sense of alienation.

The question remains, what is it in the nature of one person's relationship to herself that makes her seek out and use drugs compulsively, whereas someone else finds other means of satisfaction and self-care? Perhaps even more importantly, why is it that many people who develop abuse patterns with alcohol or drugs realize the negative effects on their lives, and moderate or quit using with little or no help from professionals or self-help groups? If we can draw a model of the internal and external factors that tend to result in serious addictive problems, we can then evaluate the treatment techniques that follow.

## Affect

By combining theory and clinical observation, psychodynamic theorists have identified a central role for affect in the development of personality. The ability to experience recognizable affect states, and to use language and fantasy to elaborate on and articulate those states, is crucial to one's sense of self. Impaired affect recognition and articulation results in difficulties with affect tolerance and modulation. If a person cannot think about an experience, he cannot give meaning to it or contain its intensity. It is this intolerance of affective experience that may be at the core of addictive problems (Morgenstern & Leeds, 1993). The technical term for such an inability to identify and articulate feelings is *alexithymia* (Krystal, 1988; Krystal & Raskin, 1970).

Joyce McDougall is well known for her work on psychosomatic disorders. She notes that whereas infants are by nature alexithymic (because they are not verbal), the development of an affective life is essential if children are to gain a sense of separate identity (McDougall, 1982). A person's private world, the internal thoughts and fantasies that are not shared with others, the sense that one is in possession of one's own body, is created by the experience and articulation of affect. Without this articulation of internal experience, an adult is vulnerable to feelings of emptiness and a tendency to express strong feelings as behavioral discharges (a small child, for instance, who is frustrated but cannot find the words to tell someone is likely to have a temper tantrum, a physical display of an emotional state). However, with members of cultures that do not share this Western value of expression of internal states, it would be a mistake to see people as exhibiting pathological behavior simply because they are reluctant to engage in a conversation regarding their innermost thoughts and feelings.

Mark and Faude (1997), using a Sullivanian interpersonal model in their work with cocaine addicts, have found that the families of cocaine-addicted patients did not talk about emotionally charged events that occurred during formative years. Physical abuse, unemployment, death, and other traumas were never discussed or processed. Such a child then grows up feeling empty or disorganized inside, with no way to modulate, express, or contain affect. This alexithymic pattern can be seen in the person's psychosocial history. Some patients may appear bland or unfeeling as they relate traumatic histories. This personality pattern makes it difficult to understand why they use drugs or alcohol at any particular time. Others display a chaotic, ruminative style of describing internal life, in which they seem aware of painful affects but have no mechanisms for modulation or articulation. In this case, their drug use is obviously linked to negative emotions.

Even without a psychodynamic orientation, a therapist can confirm by observation alone that people with serious addictive problems have great difficulty dealing with emotional experience. Whether of internal or external origin, experiences that induce strong feelings tend to be disruptive rather than just distressing to these people. Failing an important exam at school and the resulting feelings of embarrassment may cause some individuals to be overwhelmed with negative self-criticism and rush for solace. While some people go to their friends and family for support, others who cannot tolerate or articulate their distress may resort to mind-altering substances to regain their emotional equilibrium. Instead of hearing a friend say reassuring things, the person's sense of personal power and well-being is increased by the drug's effects. This type of dynamic gave rise to Khantzian's self-medication hypothesis and his attempts to pair certain drug preferences with particular affect difficulties. According to Khantzian, people who are addicted to heroin are attempting to contain and regulate aggression, whereas those who use cocaine are incapable of tolerating depressive feelings (Treece & Khantzian, 1986). Clinical observation shows that many patients with bipolar mood disorder prefer stimulants but ordinarily use them during the manic, not the depressed phase, presumably as part of an impulsive wish to intensify experiences. Paradoxically, many women who are depressed use alcohol and seem to derive some benefit from it. These are the women who, when they quit drinking, may develop a major depressive episode for the first time. Obviously, viewing the patient as actively searching for relief or assistance with affect is crucial to the understanding of addiction and the development of a treatment strategy.

## Self-Care, Self-Efficacy, and Coping Skills

Another aspect of the patient's relationship to him- or herself is behavioral in nature. While the previous sections discuss interpersonal and intrapsychic difficulties, other problems that may cause or co-occur with substance abuse disorders permeate the person's daily life in specific, concrete ways. One of the most distressing aspects of drug addiction is people's apparent lack of concern for their own well-being. A person using drugs may neglect nutrition, health problems, and personal hygiene. It is as if the drug user does not respond to the negative consequences that so bother the observer, whether a friend or therapist. These deficits come under the categories of self-care (as discussed earlier), coping skills, and self-efficacy.

Adaptive models in general hold that a person, as a result of faulty development, enters adolescence with adaptive failures. Extreme shyness, problems finishing tasks, specific learning deficits secondary to poor attention, depression, and more, may be present, causing intense distress to the individual. As young people search for ways to make up for these problems, they conduct an active search for compensatory mechanisms—people or things that can help support the weaknesses in their own makeup. If they discover drugs and alcohol as ways of coping with particular adaptive problems, and if these work well, they may become interwoven into individuals' coping styles, and, ultimately, their character structure. It is essential to understand clients' specific problems in learning and coping. For those who have already developed significant addictions, a retrospective analysis of coping strengths and weaknesses is an essential part of treatment.

Many authors discuss the importance of life skills and the dangers that face a person who has serious problems in everyday living (Marlatt & Gordon, 1985; Monti, Rohsenow, Colby, & Abrams, 1995; Peele, 1991). The clinician can make use of behavioral checklists as well as interviews to detail different problems and attempt to ascertain which of the problems predate the onset of substance use. Examples of coping skills deficits include poor communications skills, inability to resolve conflict, lack of assertiveness, lack of physical outlets for feelings, poor reading and computation skills, inability to say no to others, overwork, and poor hygiene and diet. While some of these problems may be caused by excessive use of drugs or alcohol, we should not assume that they did not exist in some form prior to the patient's drug use.

A child who has trouble paying attention in school may be suffering from attention deficit disorder or from the effects of parental discord. If the resulting difficulties with reading cause the child embarrassment, she may seek solace and a feeling of power in drug use, further interfering with her ability to learn. Obviously, the problems are not simply categorized as cause and effect of drug use. A person can have problems that contribute to the substance use as well as problems caused by it. The important point is that if a patient presents with considerable problems in different areas of coping, specific skills training such as anger management, drink refusal, or stress reduction is necessary and can be done in individual or group formats.

Finally, the *belief* that one has the ability to change is crucial to the outcome. People need to feel that they have some power over the adversity in their lives. Without a feeling of power, confidence, or self-efficacy, it is difficult to embark on, let alone continue, a course of change. The self-efficacy people experience ranges from global to specific areas of their lives. For example, Jean is a confident and articulate woman who finds her job as a sales clerk easy. Confident that she presents herself well, she can point to her sales record for confirmation of her feelings of self-efficacy in her work. In her private life, however, Jean has trouble paying her bills on time and has several creditors calling her to demand payment. She feels embarrassed and demoralized by her inability to "get it together" to pay her bills on time. Her self-efficacy in this regard is quite low. Experiences of success and failure often flow directly from variations in self-efficacy as well as actual skills levels. Throughout treatment, it is important to monitor both the patient's general feelings of self-efficacy and specific areas of confidence or lack thereof, in order to attend to shifting problem areas. A person who has quit drinking may find that he can easily say no to a drink at a friend's house (high self-efficacy) but be very worried about an upcoming wedding celebration (low self-efficacy). Understanding where the *patient* believes he is weak helps a therapist to individualize the therapy.

Working with self-efficacy and coping skills are two of the most rewarding parts of treatment. So much of psychotherapy involves painful recollections and slow progress toward healing internal wounds. Helping a person make specific, behavioral changes in a short amount of time through cognitive work and skills training is beneficial to both patient and therapist. Improved coping skills offer patients a sense of optimism and renewed commitment for the longer-term internal work that must be done.

## THE CONTRIBUTIONS OF NEUROBIOLOGY

Given the psychosocial variability of dimensions such as attachment, affect, and coping skills, it seems restrictive to think of recent advances in neurobiology and psychopharmacology as having a primary place in addiction treatment. It is just as restrictive, however, to push aside these contributions in favor of a purely psychosocial approach. Many clinicians are uncomfortable with science and embrace psychological theories as a way of avoiding new and difficult material. Others fear the encroachment of medicine on their work. Recent turf wars over prescription privileges for psychologists and biological treatments for depression, combined with the influence of the "decade of the brain" (Gabbard, 1992) in biological psychiatry, have left many clinicians, medically trained psychiatrists and psychotherapists alike, to carve out the "correct" approach for themselves, or state the basic or primary cause of psychopathologies from their own orientation. The addiction field is particularly fertile ground for such wars given the obvious biological components of addictions. Reports of the most recent research findings are often accompanied by thinking that equates correlation with causation. Just because a person may carry a gene and end up an alcoholic does not mean that the gene *caused* the alcohol problem. In another way, just because a person had an unhappy childhood does not mean that we can say that this is the cause of later alcohol problems. Many factors are associated, or correlated, with alcohol and drug problems (Kranzler & Anton, 1997). Those who insist on finding a purely biological or psychological cause are doomed to disappointment, and they doom the rest of us to inadequate treatment models.

The explosion of research on reward centers (Gardner, 1997) and brain changes makes it almost impossible to offer a coherent perspective on this topic. New information suggesting that the neurotransmitter dopamine is responsible for "the rush" or the reward following ingestion of a psychoactive drug leads to speculation about possible medications to block this effect, thereby reducing the attractiveness (physiologically) of drugs. Other studies indicate the low levels of dopamine $D_2$ receptors in the brain may cause an increase in the pleasure response to psychostimulants. Such findings suggest that increasing dopamine receptor levels might also counter the reward aspects of stimulant use (Volkow et al., 1999). Indications of changes in actual brain structure as a result of trauma point to the inescapable interaction of experience and physiology. The variable roles of genetic determinism, environmental correlates, trauma, and chemical insult resulting from repeated drug use are impossible to separate. Practitioners are likely either to reject scientific information as irrelevant or incomprehensible, or to cling to different studies as evidence of their most cherished beliefs. This polarization is unnecessary given that the research supports an interactive, biopsychosocial approach, despite some people's efforts to advertise the finding of an absolute cause or cure for addiction.

Genetic research provides us with an example of this dilemma. We tend to think of genetic influences on an individual as being permanent. Genes carry the information for how the body makes itself and how it repairs damage. We do not think that we can alter our genetic heritage after birth. It is more accurate, however, to think of genes as a blueprint that can be altered by many mechanisms, both chemical and experiential. Changes in the basic building blocks of our body, DNA, may be more difficult to affect by life experiences, but messenger RNA (contained in brain nerve cells) is clearly responsive to chemical influences such as antidepressant medications (Stahl,

1996). The brain changes that are caused by negative experiences, primarily those in childhood, do in fact result in genetic changes via the messenger RNA system. Thus, the brain can be permanently altered by one's emotional life early in childhood or by intense experiences as an adult (Schore, 1994).

Those in the field of neurobiology are discovering and positing theories about the interaction among biological systems, experience, and the ultimate structure and functions of the brain. Some of the findings are amazing and exciting; others are frightening in their implications for individual development. Work in areas such as pleasure and reward systems, attachment, stress, and trauma reveal an interrelatedness that makes the term "biopsychosocial" come to life with intense force. This section outlines important information from these research areas and suggests possible interactions for use in the assessment and treatment of addictive disorders.

## The Neurobiology of Attachment

People typically develop strong attachments to others. As clinicians, we often see patients whose attachments are fraught with conflict and confusion, or absent altogether. Often, we wonder what could possibly bind one person to another given the details of their painful interactions. Why is it that abused children maintain loyalty to the parent who is hurting them? Why do adults cling to relationships that are abusive in some way? Of course, there are many psychological theories to account for this, but the strength and universality of attachment behavior indicates the presence of underlying biological factors as well. Bowlby (1982) asserts that people, like other animals, are hardwired to form attachments or bonds. In children, any threat of separation elicits a stress response, a cry, or a motor expression intended to bring the mother back. Adults have a complementary response toward the young. Both child and adult strive to protect the bond by maintaining proximity to one another. The benefits for infant survival are obvious. Less obvious, but just as important, these bonds are reinforced by trauma, even if suffered at the hands of the primary caretaker. The three types of attachment bonds—secure, anxious, and avoidant (Ainsworth, Blehar, Waters, & Wall, 1978)—have physiological correlates that are only now being identified through animal and human research.

Insel's (1997) studies on pair bonding and parental behavior in mammals offer intriguing information regarding the workings of brain chemicals on complex social behaviors. The neuropeptides oxytocin and vasopressin were thought to be endocrine hormones, manufactured in the brain but delivered to organs in the body far from the brain. Insel's research suggests that these peptides are also neurotransmitters that have direct action in the brain, particularly in the limbic system, the region of the brain known for its relationship to human emotions and social behavior. Dopamine, also a neurotransmitter with actions in this brain region, is known to affect maternal behavior in animals as well as emotions in humans. If these chemical systems are disrupted, whether by genetic anomaly, brain insult, or experience, significant problems in attachment may be more likely to develop. Without the bonds between self and others, behaviors that appear antisocial are more likely, and the ability to care for oneself could also conceivably be impaired.

## Affect Regulation and Emotional Development

Researchers working in the area of early childhood brain development are gaining insight into the interaction between life experiences and brain development (Schore, 1994, 1996). Affective life and attachment bonds are interwoven for the young child, most critically in the first 2 years of life. During this time, attachment experiences control and affect the alterations of several important brain chemicals: opioids, corticosteroids (stress hormones), and peptides, as discussed earlier. These chemicals in turn control how the brain develops important connections, or neural pathways, that will determine to a large extent the expression of affect and the development of attachment styles. The changes that occur are hardwired into the developing brain and serve to mediate emotional life throughout the lifespan. It is through the interaction of attachment experiences and brain physiology that the dopamine, serotonin, and norepinephrine systems mature. These neurotransmitters are implicated in the expression of psychiatric symptoms and affected by antidepressant and antipsychotic medications. It appears that distressful experiences in early childhood, most notably *repeated*, *chronic* experiences of emotional distress, leave the young person with an emotional system that is both permanently reactive and underdeveloped.

One example of this complex interaction is the gazing that takes place between mother and child. The face is a source of emotional information to us. As the infant brain begins to process visual information, the infant's experience of gazing at the mother's face, if the gaze is returned with positive emotion, releases large amounts of dopamine and endorphins. These chemicals are known to be related to the experience of pleasure, pain relief, and satisfaction, and are the major chemicals implicated in the "rush" or the "high" of drug use. The implications are clear. If a child is stressed by the lack of positive emotional experiences, the brain will not set down pathways for dopamine and endorphins, possibly resulting in a person who cannot experience pleasure or find ways to soothe the self during difficult times. Some of these people will eventually show signs of emotional disturbance, behavioral dysfunction, and addiction.

## Trauma

Much of the research and clinical speculation about early experience and its effects on brain development centers around the issue of trauma. The field is too extensive to review in this book, and the separation of trauma from general emotional development is an arbitrary one. First of all, trauma is not necessarily the result of one acute episode of negative experience. Trauma can be inflicted by consistent negative events that may be subthreshold for the immediate expression of any response. For example, children who are consistently ignored when asking for attention may not show, or experience consciously, significant distress. Over time, however, the effects of this treatment become evident: One child begins to act out in order to bring attention to himself; another child withdraws. Cultural biases in child-rearing practices, such as described by Walant (1995), sometimes result in parental behavior that give the child what she calls experiences of "normative abuse," emotionally damaging experiences that most people would not see as traumatic because they result from a culturally sanctioned parenting mode. Spanking is one good example of normative abuse. This practice is not as acceptable as it once was, but 20 years ago, no one would have considered it to be traumatic for the child; it was merely formative.

Of course, some children *do* experience intense physical, sexual, and verbal abuse. The effects of this type of abuse, if consistent, can overwhelm the emotional capacities of the child and lead to permanent derangement of various brain systems. The work of van der Kolk, McFarlane, and Weisaeth (1996) provides a chilling look into the neurobiology of trauma. In general, van der Kolk suggests that trauma leads to a biphasic response in the brain, characterized by hyperresponsivity followed by numbing. The brain chemicals involved are dopamine, norepinephrine, and serotonin. During acute stress, the brain is flooded with norepinephrine (just as the body is flooded by adrenaline during the fight–flight response). It reacts with a constellation of physiological hyperresponses that eventually lead to depletion of dopamine, norepinephrine, and serotonin, causing various psychological and behavioral symptoms. The initial response results in intrusive symptoms, such as recurring thoughts of the trauma, or in general hyperarousal, including an exaggerated startle response. These symptoms persist because the stress of long-term hyperarousal leads to depletion of norepinephrine and dopamine. The second part of the biphasic response to stress includes symptoms such as emotional numbing, deficits in learning, decreased motivation, and emotional constriction. Additionally, it is thought that the aggressiveness and impulsivity often seen in victims of trauma are related to serotonin depletion (caused by the body's incapacity to synthesize more serotonin quickly enough to counteract the effects of ongoing stress; low levels of serotonin are associated with aggression).

In earlier work, van der Kolk (1988) has shown that pain and traumatic stress cause a stress-induced analgesia (SIA) as a result of the release of endogenous opiates in the brain. Chronic overproduction of these narcotic-like brain chemicals can result in a dependence and withdrawal cycle that resembles heroin and morphine addiction (van der Kolk, 1988). The implications for the possible origins of narcotic addiction are obvious. While it is easy to see the connection between early childhood trauma and narcotic addiction, what is less clear is the role that narcotics play in *causing* a depletion cycle and whether the depletion is permanent. This chicken-and-egg scenario, interesting for research, is important for clinicians because it may help explain relapse from a biological standpoint, and may move us toward pharmacotherapies for certain addictions. Currently, pharmacotherapy stresses the use of blocking agents, chemicals that cause the brain to not respond to the pleasurable effects of certain drugs of abuse. Only methadone treatment attempts to actually *replace* a drug of abuse with one that has similar effects. Of course, societal attitudes regarding drug use affect clinical decisions about how we help people with drug problems. Will we allow substitute drugs to relieve emotional pain, or will we concentrate most on drugs that block the pleasure of drug use?

## Brain Reward Mechanisms

The idea of mimicking or blocking drug effects in the brain by the use of medications is based on a new understanding of the role that certain drugs play in producing pleasure. Current research points to dopamine as being responsible for the experience of the rush or high associated with the use of psychoactive drugs such as alcohol, nicotine, cocaine, and heroin. Researchers and the press are popularizing the notion that addiction may be caused by a deficit in dopamine production or a lack of sensitivity to it (e.g., Nash, 1997; Nestler, 1995). What seems to be true is that all psychoactive drugs affect dopamine in a number of different ways (Stahl, 1996). These effects are only just beginning to be discovered. Cocaine apparently blocks the reabsorption (reuptake) of dopamine, resulting in more of the chemical staying active, producing a continuous effect. Amphetamines also disable the reuptake of dopamine, with the same effect of increasing the amount and activity of dopamine on the synapse. Nicotine acts to stimulate the release of dopamine, but nicotine also appears to block the action of an enzyme, monoamine oxidase, that usually breaks down dopamine, allowing the neurotransmitter to remain in the synapse for longer than usual.

The mechanism is less clear, but depressant drugs such as alcohol and heroin also affect the release of dopamine in the brain. Pleasure and feelings of contentment and well-being are potent reinforcers. It is no wonder that drugs have such appeal in general. This may help explain why people whose brains have been affected by negative childhood experiences might find drugs so compelling. Do these people lack adequate internal brain reward systems and use drugs to replace what is missing biochemically, or do they use drugs to gain a sense of pleasure in a life otherwise devoid of it? The answer is probably a complex interaction of these and other forces, with variations from individual to individual. Eventually, knowledge of these mechanisms might allow us to plan treatment interventions accordingly. People whose brains seem to be permanently damaged would benefit more in the short run from medication to replace ill-functioning brain structures than from insight-oriented psychotherapy. With all the research on brain mechanisms, it is easy to forget that by the time people come to treatment, their use of drugs is interwoven into their character, defenses, and lifestyle, and is no longer (if it ever was) a simple product of brain chemistry. Multiple and parallel interventions will prove most effective in the long run.

# CHAPTER FIVE

# Clinical Cases Using Harm Reduction Psychotherapy

**W**hile it is important to consider many complex and competing factors when designing treatment for people with drug and alcohol problems, it is, after all, the relationship between the patient and therapist that will prove therapeutic. This important element cannot be adequately conveyed in isolation from case material. Rather than describe in detail the many types of treatment approaches from which one can choose, this chapter consists entirely of case studies designed to allow the reader to see treatment in action. Supporting information regarding specific treatment interventions (cognitive-behavioral, relapse prevention, self-help, etc.) is contained in Appendix F.

## THE CASE OF JOAN (Continued)

Joan, the woman whose case was highlighted earlier, continued in treatment with me for 1 year. Her therapy was designed to take into account the multitude of problems with which she came into treatment, including her unwillingness to explore childhood experiences.

This case, as well as the others in this chapter, contains background information, so that the reader can see the treatment plan as it developed. Background information and assessment results are followed by a focus on central clinical issues and themes, as well as any special considerations. The treatment plans include the patients' hierarchy of needs and goals, and the course of treatment includes references to models developed by other clinicians as well as by myself. Finally, the outcome of treatment is presented with commentary.

Joan was 27 years old at the time she entered therapy. She was upset about a pattern of unstable relationships and showed clear signs of other instability as well. The loss of her parents, her subsequent stay in the orphanage where her brother committed suicide, and where she was abused, and the later drinking relationship with her grandmother all contributed to these significant problems. The results of the assessment (MAP), which took about eight sessions over a 2-month period to complete, indicated that a multifaceted psychotherapy would be necessary to address her problems and that her prognosis was questionable. She had no stable support system within the lesbian community and very little self-efficacy for change. The most immediate problematic clinical issue was her intense fear of, and reaction to, experiences that felt to her like abandonment. At those times, her general inability to modulate and tolerate affect resulted in outbursts of jealousy and unreasonable demands on others. These outbursts were punctuated by self-injurious behaviors that threatened to compromise her health and life, as well as her therapy. I was particularly concerned by her use of cocaine intravenously. She would shoot up repeatedly for hours, using large amounts over a short period of time, which produced on her arms severe abscesses that required medical attention. Such a use pattern, especially given that her other drug use, while extensive, was not particularly dangerous, marked her intravenous use as having particular symbolic meaning for her.

The fact that Joan became acutely suicidal when she did attempt to abstain from drugs and alcohol was an ominous sign, indicating a serious underlying depression that, given her impulsivity, was very likely to put her at risk for acting on those suicidal feelings. Such an intense suicidal reaction also indicated the importance of Joan's attachment to these drugs, such that the loss of them plunged her into despair. Clearly, the alcohol and drugs had become her primary support system. She had tried using 12-Step meetings as a substitute attachment, but she could not make the leap. In order for the therapy to progress with minimal danger to Joan, I had to make some accommodation to this fact.

Joan expressed great reluctance to explore any childhood experiences, becoming quite tearful and agitated if I pursued anything but the most superficial questions. Conducting the kind of in-depth psychotherapy that she needed was going to be difficult given this restriction. The one positive indicator was that Joan seemed to like me and was able to tell me when to back off with my questions. She used her charms to engage me, starting and ending each session with some cute remark or look that could only be construed as seductive. I chose to view this as her way of making a connection that she desperately needed, so I made no comment but expressed to her that I felt hopeful about our work together.

Often, the complete hierarchy of needs in a case such as Joan's cannot at first be detailed. She was in considerable distress, acted out with potentially dangerous behaviors, and had obvious need of containment. She desperately wanted to feel some relief as soon as possible. The first need, then, was to make a plan to change one part of her behavior quickly. This would accomplish both some measure of containment and relieve some of her distress. The second priority, working with her jealousy in relationships, would have to wait until Joan experienced some behavioral success with her drug or alcohol use.

Joan and I constructed an initial treatment plan that was graduated and detailed. I did not insist that we talk about her childhood, but I did let her know that I could not imagine resolving her problems with relationships without some exploration of early experiences. Nor did I insist that she had to change something immediately regarding her drug use; rather, I had her agree that it would be useful to explore the connections between her drug use, her behavior, and her feelings. With these caveats, we began treatment in earnest. Since she was in the contemplation stage of change regarding both her drug use and participation in treatment, I first focused her attention on a decisional balance, allowing her to express all sides of her ambivalence about her relationship to drugs. I was able to establish clear connections between her excessive use of alcohol and fights with her girlfriend, so that Joan became interested in decreasing her use of this substance. To accomplish this, I used a new harm reduction method called substance use management. This strategy, loosely based on Hester and Miller's (1989) behavioral self-control training, is designed to decrease tolerance to alcohol and moderate the amount and timing of drinks. Joan agreed to measure her drinks for a few days, so that we could establish a baseline. She was averaging eight drinks per day, all of them between the hours of 6:00 P.M. and 2:00 A.M. I suggested that she decrease the number of drinks by one each day for a week, then stay at one or two drinks per day for another week. After this period, she was to drink no more than four drinks and only between the hours of 8:00 P.M. and midnight. This would decrease her tolerance, reduce her total alcohol intake, and restrict the intrusion of drinking into her environment, so that other things might have a chance to take its place. Joan was unable to reduce her drinking below four drinks a day in that first week, but she felt proud of herself for doing that much. She saw it as an indication that she could exert control without causing great emotional distress, and I saw it as a step in the right direction, as well as an important experience of self-efficacy for Joan. The emphasis on "any positive change" is crucial to harm reduction psychotherapy.

One evening, Joan exceeded her drinking limit by many drinks and got into a fight with her new girlfriend. She was able to see that alcohol played a role in intensifying her feelings and rendering her more out of control. From that time on, she rarely exceeded her limit, although she did not decrease her use. Interestingly, she changed her drinking pattern on the evenings when she came to therapy. About 10 weeks into the therapy, I noticed that she smelled of alcohol when she arrived, and her fair skin was flushed. She explained that she was using two of her four drinks that night to calm herself down enough to come into my office. She felt certain that it would help her talk in a more open way, but mostly she felt she needed it to calm her intense anticipatory anxiety. Although I had avoided the most loaded topics of her childhood, I could not avoid making some links. In order to help her to manage her anxiety, I added specific affect tolerance work to the therapeutic work. While she was interested in a good outcome, she was not very engaged in the process, wanting to spend her time talking about how to deal with her girlfriend, so she would not be left again. The work I suggested was that she focus on a feeling that she had just expressed or felt in the session and expand on it verbally. I then asked her to rate the feeling on a scale of 1 to 10 related to how it compared with the same feeling at other times. Next, I asked her to visualize this rating scale as a dial and to slowly move the dial down one notch, from 8 to 7, for example. I taught her how to use her brain rather than her body or her feelings to conduct this exercise. She found it useful at the moment but had little interest in pursuing the exercise on her own. Since I could not get her to focus on the meaning of her feelings, we were stuck with lackluster results in the area of affect tolerance.

The most significant breakthrough occurred after she had spent an entire weekend shooting cocaine intravenously. She was very upset with herself and worried that she had done some permanent nerve damage. Now, for the first time, Joan was interested in figuring out *why* she did this. Although I was careful not to offer any suggestions to her, Joan was able to realize that her use of powder cocaine and intravenous cocaine were two very different behaviors and experiences, motivated by different internal states. Her use of powder cocaine was always a recreational event, shared with friends within the context of a social scene while dancing or talking at bars. But she always used intravenous cocaine alone. No one knew that she shot coke. Why would she need to do this? After a couple of sessions, Joan had noticed that when she was experiencing some vague but intense sense of discomfort or depression, she was using cocaine intravenously. Noting that shooting up made her feel even worse, I asked her if she was trying to hurt herself by doing this. She responded to my question with one of those "deer in the headlights" stares and nodded "yes." She looked and felt stunned for a few moments but then began talking about wanting to die all the time and how drugs and alcohol usually made her forget that. She also said that it was the same feeling that she had as a kid in the orphanage, and she related this to her brother's suicide. I labeled her use of intravenous cocaine as a suicide attempt and she agreed. We made a plan for her to contact me when she felt the urge to shoot up. She did this several times over the next few months. It was one of the few indications that Joan was allowing herself to use me as a supportive relationship.

Joan continued to come to therapy weekly but would not agree to come more often when I suggested it to her. She stopped drinking before sessions, and also discontinued drinking every night. She developed a pattern of drinking only when she was alone, since she realized that she could have fun socially without it and got into less trouble interpersonally when she was sober. She continued to insist that she needed the alcohol other times, and I labeled it her "antidepressant," suggesting that perhaps we could find a better antidepressant for her at a pharmacy. She refused, saying that she was trying not to use drugs regularly and did not want to add another one to the mix. This logic is typical of drug and alcohol users, who will use various substances of unknown quality but are very reluctant to take antidepressants. In their perception, drug use is generally under their control. The intentional use of drugs to create an effect gives them a much-needed feeling of being able to intervene positively in their own distress. Antidepressant medications cannot be used in this intermittent, as-needed manner, and are thus not seen as useful. I interpreted Joan's reluctance as her wanting to be in charge of her medications and titrate the dose to the desired effect. She agreed, but I could not persuade her that a more stable pharmacological effect might also even out her moods and impulses. Ordinarily, I would have pursued this topic more aggressively, since antidepressant medications often can help decrease depression even while a person continues drinking. These medications can also help a person cut down or quit drug use altogether by interfering with craving. This anti-craving factor, particularly in the drug Wellbutrin, which has recently been relicensed under the name Zyban for smoking cessation, is creating optimism about the development of specific pharmacological interventions for cravings and withdrawal symptoms. However, Joan was also taking stimulants, which do not mix well with most antidepressants, and she had narcotics in her system as well. I reluctantly agreed with her that another drug might not be what she needed most.

Joan continued to moderate her drug use and had only one more episode of suicidal intravenous cocaine use during the year. She was more able to control her anger and jealousy with girlfriends and her work continued to go well. She had made only modest gains in terms of tolerating her feelings of pain and sadness, and she did not want to talk about them. Her avoidance strategy was beginning to interfere with the therapy because she no longer had the "loud" symptoms to offer as our focus.

Joan's therapy came to an abrupt end after 1 year, when I moved my office from San Francisco to Oakland, across the Bay Bridge. She flatly stated that she was terrified of crossing the bridge and would also not ride the subway underneath the bay. After several weeks of discussing plans to reduce her fear, we set up an appointment at the new office that she never kept, calling from the bus station to say that she was too frightened. She missed her next appointment and did not call, nor did she ever return my calls to her.

Needless to say, this type of termination leaves the therapist bewildered and, in my case, sad and guilty as well. I believe that once Joan's worst symptoms stabilized, she could no longer avoid facing the events of her childhood and the intense feelings and depression associated with it. She knew also that she would have to make even more dramatic changes in her drug and alcohol use. Whatever attachment she had forged with me was not strong enough, or was too threatening, to anchor her through that process. Perhaps our relationship had reactivated her fears of abandonment. I have spent much time wondering what I might have done differently and whether it would have actually made a difference. Creating a more intense therapeutic relationship might have given her the security she needed to pursue her painful work, but at the risk of increasing her fears of abandonment. The balance between too much and too little closeness in the therapeutic relationship is tenuous with patients who have suffered so much early loss and trauma.

## SPEED AND SEX: THE CASE OF DAN

Dan was 36 years old, single, and, at the time he began therapy, a sales manager for a local business machines company. He had a bachelor's degree in business administration. He was referred to me by a friend who saw my brochure in his therapist's waiting room. Dan vaguely said that he had a drug problem but was reluctant to give details, nor did he indicate what exactly he wanted to do about the problem. Dan was also experiencing severe money problems despite his excellent abilities to manage his company's money. He appeared shy and anxious, and made no eye contact with me. While Dan had had no previous therapy experience, he had gone to Narcotics Anonymous (NA) meetings several times over the past year but did not like the group format or the idea that he would have to admit that he was powerless. He had tried to make use of the program, however, and had contacted a sponsor, but they "didn't really click." He gave few other details. His family history was sketchy. Dan said only that his mother and father stayed together for the sake of the three children, but no one really talked much or got along. He had been married when he was 20, but divorced within 2 years because he "liked to have sex with other people, too."

Despite my attempts to adhere to the principles of motivational interviewing, such as asking only open-ended questions, the style turned into a question-and-answer format because of Dan's guardedness. I was unable to interest Dan in examining his reluctance to talk, and the more I tried to focus on our process, the more non-communicative he became. I was very uncomfortable with the style of our interaction but proceeded with information gathering, looking for any hint that he might prefer a shift to a more interactive format. Of course, clarifying goals was equally difficult. Even though Dan said that he wanted to quit using drugs, he could not articulate any good reasons to quit, or reasons that he continued to use, for that matter. Because of his interest in focusing on his drug use, he appeared to be in the contemplation stage of change. I was blocked, however, from using the primary intervention for that stage, the decisional balance, because of his inability to talk about his experience.

Speed was Dan's drug of choice, although he also abused alcohol in concert with the speed. His pattern was very specific. He did not use during the week, postponing any urges until weekends or when away on business trips. He would go out to a club or a bar after injecting methamphetamine (crystal meth) and begin drinking to take the edge off. He would pick up somebody and go to a hotel, where they would have sex repeatedly and continue to use speed and alcohol together. These episodes, sometimes with multiple partners, often lasted until early Monday morning, when he would return home and get ready for the work week. After it became apparent that he was avoiding the mention of any partner's name or gender, I asked him how many of his partners were male. (I used this phrase, *how many*, rather than *are any*, which is the best way to ask sexual history questions because it does not allow a "yes" or "no" answer and communicates to the person the therapist's understanding that many people have sex with a partner of the same gender). He paused so long that I thought he had not heard my question. After a while, he quietly answered, "Yes," then lapsed into an uncomfortable silence, not meeting my eyes, but glancing up to see my reaction. I chose to avoid any comment or question and proceeded with a business-like attitude. It is not typical for me to be so avoidant of process or exploration with a patient, but Dan's demeanor felt like a barrier and a warning for me to keep my professional distance.

In terms of the level of abuse, he was clearly abusing both speed and alcohol but appeared to have no physical dependence on either. Because of his compulsive preoccupation, an inability to stop using once the binge had begun, and sexual practices that could have serious negative consequences, he met the criteria for substance dependence, a more serious disorder than abuse.

Dan had no social networks. His parents lived in another state and he had little contact with them or with his older brother or younger sister. He was a loner, who rarely went out with coworkers and had no close friends except for one old college roommate who lived in the area. This friend was aware of Dan's drug problem and had offered to help in any way he could, but Dan could not think of any way his friend could be of help and was, in fact, ashamed of himself for the fact that he "blurted out" his problem one morning when he was recuperating from a weekend binge. There was no history of previous psychiatric intervention. Dan had never sought help for any emotional or behavioral problems. Other than his drug problem, he did not at first appear to have any diagnosable mental condition, although his extreme aloofness and social isolation made me think of either schizoid or avoidant traits, if not a clear personality disorder. He did feel suicidal at times, but this occurred only after binges and did not appear to be part of a depressive disorder.

The clinical issues and themes were evident from the beginning. Emotional isolation, shame about sexual behaviors, and an inability to communicate with others or form attachments made Dan a difficult person with whom to initiate contact and a poor candidate for insight-oriented therapy. These issues also created a solid platform for the creation of drug dependence. One of the difficulties was that, while Dan obviously needed assistance with his drug problem, he was very wary of allowing any person to know him too well. I decided to find a way of acting as a consultant to him rather than a therapist, hoping to establish a business-type relationship that would allow him to remain distant yet still take advantage of my help. I made use of some of the concepts and techniques of solution-focused treatment (Berg & Miller, 1992; see Appendix F) to engage Dan in this collaborative relationship. For example, I stressed whatever small changes he made as evidence that he was not stuck but had already been successful at changing his use. I also referred often to his abilities to make plans and execute them.

Dan readily agreed that he wanted to stop using speed and alcohol, but was afraid that he could not maintain sobriety in the face of the intense cravings he experienced. As he described these cravings, it became clear that what he called "drug cravings" were actually a final series of feelings, most notably loneliness and sexual tension. I did not think, however, that he was ready to deal with these feelings. I helped Dan focus on his most identifying trigger for using, the approaching weekends. The strategies I employed were supportive and educational in nature. I suggested several alternative self-help books for him to read (see Appendix D), and coached him through the exercises in a workbook (Horvath, 1998). I offered matter-of-fact support and encouragement and responded to his successes and failures with little display of emotion. Even though Dan was not consistently meeting his goal of abstinence, I decided that the relapse prevention methods (Marlatt & Gordon, 1985) of educating him and structuring his response to cravings and triggers might work well. This involved identifying specific, high-risk situations and developing several coping strategies that could be employed at such times.

Dan used speed on two weekends immediately after beginning treatment. We discussed the buildup of tension that he felt, starting on the previous Wednesdays, as he looked forward to the weekend and relaxation. These thoughts quickly led to a compulsive preoccupation with whether he would use drugs and an intense internal debate, during which he would berate himself for being weak. I convinced him to practice thought stopping when the internal arguments began and to do one of the exercises in the book instead. I avoided interpreting what I viewed as his superego conflicts and the punitive nature of his internal world, which necessitated rebellion. The link between his speed use and sex clearly revealed this dynamic. Whether or not Dan was actually gay, he had intense negative feelings about his sexual urges toward men and could only indulge in them when in an altered state. These issues probably got in the way of long-term sobriety, but this was not the time to explore them. I also suggested that he find an NA group that was very large and not use a sponsor, but he did not want to do that again. I suggested this because the NA format offers a specific, behavioral program that could supplement the work he and I were doing. In addition, by going to a large meeting and not having a sponsor, Dan could avoid the interpersonal contact that made him so uneasy in his therapy with me.

After attending sessions for about 4 months, Dan quit using speed for 3 months but had little to say during these subsequent sessions. He decided to quit therapy, and I could offer no reason for him to continue, since he did not appear to feel the need for support and clearly did not want to talk about anything more intimate. Dan contacted me after about 6 months to say that he had joined an NA group that was large enough that he did not have to talk. He had been clean for 4 months and had not engaged in anonymous sex during that time.

I was happy for Dan. Apparently the one-on-one contact was too much for him, but he could not do the initial work on his own. He used me to get started on a self-help program, eventually finding a way to give himself the structure that a program without much interpersonal contact could provide.

## SELF-ESTEEM, MOTIVATION, AND CRACK: THE CASE OF ANGIE

Angie, a 24-year-old African American dental hygienist, had worked at the same job for 3 years while she attended a local college. She hoped to be a lawyer some day: "If I can ever get my shit together." She chose my name out of an insurance panel list because my office was "in a nice neighborhood, . . . far away from [her] downtown office." She was direct and articulate, stating that she had been addicted to crack for over a year, and it was beginning to take a toll on her work, her studies, but most importantly, her self-esteem. She grew up with a younger brother and sister in Southern California, moving to Chicago when she was 12. Her father was a college professor, and her mother worked as a part-time fund-raiser for political campaigns. Both parents were heavy drinkers at different points in her life, but Angie was unaware of any drug use by either of them. They divorced when Angie was 17, and she split her time between them.

Angie had moved to the San Francisco Bay area 4 years earlier to be with a boyfriend she had met while on vacation. She had never used drugs or alcohol before she met him, believing that drugs were sure to be an impediment to her life goals. She also expressed disdain for men she had met who wanted her to be pretty but not smart, referring especially to this previous boyfriend. He introduced her to marijuana, which she used only twice because it made her "want to eat the entire kitchen," and to crack cocaine. Angie enjoyed the high that she got from crack and smoked it with her friends on weekends before going out dancing. She also liked the way it took away her appetite, as she was very conscious of her body and wanted to "keep it tight." After she and her boyfriend broke up, however, Angie started using crack by herself to ward off feelings of depression and loneliness. She was able to control her use to a few pipes several times per week for many months, but in the previous 6-month period, she had been using large quantities every day, often going into work without having slept at all. Aware that her work was suffering, she was worried that her boss would notice. Also ashamed of what she saw as her own weakness, Angie wanted to quit using all together.

Angie mentioned that she might like a group of other women similar to herself. What she meant by this was a group of middle-class black women. She was struggling with a difficult split both within herself, and between herself and the black community. She had grown up middle class in a predominantly white neighborhood. She felt ashamed of the poverty and self-destruction that she encountered in many of her current black neighbors who had grown up differently. While she couched her statements carefully, she was clearly trying to develop an identity as a black woman while harboring strong internalized racism. I saw her wish for a group as a desire for support in this difficult developmental task.

Angie, who showed clear signs of cocaine dependence, was in the preparation stage of change. She was clear about the negative consequences, both present and future, of her crack use and could see no reason to continue even though she found it hard even to try quitting. She had had no previous therapy and showed no obvious signs of depression, anxiety, or a personality disorder. At most, she had developed an adjustment disorder after breaking up with her boy-friend. She had a wide group of friends, including several close fe-male friends and a few close male friends. Her girlfriends were aware of her cocaine addiction, but she did not really talk to anyone about it in great depth. Angie's younger sister was a crack addict living in poverty, a fact of which she was ashamed and a situation she was de-termined to avoid.

This seemed to be a straightforward case of a goal-oriented, high-functioning woman who was struggling primarily with the physiological addictive properties of crack cocaine. I recommended outpatient therapy once per week. This had no impact after 1 month, and Angie was becoming concerned. She thought that she first needed something much more structured to help her break the habit. Despite the fact that she did not particularly want to take the time off from work, she agreed to a 2-week inpatient program, followed by 6 months of aftercare outpatient treatment. The expense of this pro-gram was such that she could only afford to see me once per month. We focused on supporting abstinence and practicing drug-refusal skills. Angie also talked a lot about her career aspirations and her de-termination to move forward as quickly as possible. After 3 months, Angie decided to quit the outpatient follow-up program because she could not stand all the "powerless crap" and all the people who were relapsing. She also did not like being told that she could not drink al-cohol despite the fact that she drank only a glass or two of wine about once per month. She felt that she knew more about herself than the people in the program, who would not listen to her. She found herself withholding information in order to avoid confronta-tions but did not feel good about that. She agreed to return to ther-apy once per week; we talked about the dangers of increased alcohol use to compensate for lack of crack. She agreed that if her drinking increased, she would monitor her drinks by writing in a journal and talking to me about it.

Angie maintained abstinence from crack for the next 5 months and experienced few cravings. Luckily, there was no increase in her alcohol use. Interestingly, she was quite prepared to quit drinking if she saw herself beginning to use more, and she used this as a "gentle threat" to herself whenever she considered taking a drink more often than once or twice per month. Angie terminated therapy after a total of 8 months. She calls occasionally to let me know that she is doing fine. Before she left therapy, she found a young professional women's support group, where she began to discuss her racial identity. She continues to find this helpful.

Angie, who clearly knew what she wanted and how to get there, is a good example of maturing out of an addiction (Peele, 1991), a process of growing up to find that drug use interferes with one's goals in life. Angie also had the additional motivation of seeing her sister ruin her life with drugs. Because of her good ego strength, she was also determined to be a strong black woman and defy the cultural stereotypes of the single-mother drug addict. Angie represents young women who are often introduced to drugs by their boyfriends and either cannot say no or are initially as enamored of the drug as they are of the boyfriend. Early intervention and assertiveness training skills are important for these young women in this society.

## LOST IN AMERICA: THE CASE OF ZEKE

Zeke, a 31-year-old white male nurse, worked in an inpatient ward and had a long history of drug use. He was referred to me by a colleague who knew him socially. He agreed to come only because this person had assured him that I would listen to *his* perception of his life and not assume that I knew what was best for him. Zeke was worried because his current narcotics habit was out of control. At the time, he mostly used heroin. His usual supplier had moved, and he had stolen some morphine from work on two occasions. Afraid that he would get caught, Zeke was not sure that he could stop himself. He was also experiencing intense frustration at work and had recently had a couple of "blowups."

Zeke had used intravenous heroin and smoked opium while traveling in Asia for several years in his late teens, but after quitting for over 8 years, he had started using again 2 years previously. During that time, he often drank heavily but was more interested in psychedelics and marijuana. Despite his regular heavy use of alcohol and marijuana, Zeke put himself through a B.A. nursing program and had been working steadily since graduation. He had worked in the emergency room but did not like the frenetic pace, tried pediatrics but found working with sick children too distressing, and finally settled in a surgical position that he felt suited his temperament.

Zeke's upbringing was the key to understanding both his drug use and his complaints of boredom and dissatisfaction with life. Born and raised on a commune in Arizona, he was raised by an ever-changing assortment of adults and in the company of many children. While knowing that his mother and father loved him, he always felt shy and unsure of himself and was painfully aware of his parents' limitations in terms of guidance or advice. Both parents "smoked a lot of pot," and after their divorce, when Zeke was 12, his father moved to Northern California and became a large-scale marijuana grower. During the school year, Zeke lived with his mother, who moved around a lot, and he found it difficult to establish new friend-ships. He spent summers with his father and his new commune friends. Zeke had always felt that other people were great and inter-esting but not of much use when he was trying to figure out who he was and how to live. He married a childhood friend at age 20, but she left him the following year because of his drug use. This event had precipitated his quitting narcotics at that time.

At the point of intake, Zeke was physically dependent on intra-venous heroin, which he supplemented with opium that he grew him-self. He was also smoking marijuana daily, but he had quit drinking alcohol a month prior to entering treatment. He did this because it was his least favorite drug and he wanted to get a head start on the process of changing himself. Despite this action, his goals were un-clear. Zeke was in the contemplation stage of change and appeared to have been stuck there for a long time despite his preparatory ef-forts. It occurred to me that his long-term use of marijuana might be contributing to his vagueness about treatment goals. Zeke also was in need of an attachment figure who, unlike his parents, could offer some clear guidance and "be of use" to him. I decided to recommend individual therapy for Zeke and used my understanding of attach-ment theory to design interventions.

It was not at all clear to Zeke what he wanted out of therapy. He expressed an awareness that it was time for him to do "some serious looking at myself again," and he said that previous therapy experi-ences had been very useful. All of these therapies had been expres-sive, New Age–types of programs conducted mostly in group format. He was intrigued at my suggestion that we *just talk*. After I explained the nature of "talk therapy" and the therapeutic relationship, Zeke became very quiet. He said that no one had ever seemed really to want to connect with him, and he did not quite get how that would help, nor did he trust that I might actually want to help him. This session identified the main therapeutic theme and barrier that would permeate his treatment. Zeke had never been able to count on any-one to provide concrete guidance in a nurturing, structured format. He had grown up under a benevolent surveillance that offered little structure and people who had no expectations of him. As an adult, he was always dissatisfied with his life even though he did not think there was anything particularly wrong with it.

Zeke was open about his drug history and seemed proud of it as well. He felt that drugs, especially marijuana and the psychedelics, gave him a perspective on people and the world that helped make him a good person. At the same time, he knew that his narcotic ad-diction was interfering with his ability to enter into social or intimate relationships. Since he was ambivalent about relationships anyway, his motivation to quit was not very sturdy. Zeke felt that he alone had to make and carry out the decision to quit. It had never occurred to him that someone might be able to help him sort out his feelings and make some decisions about his drug use, without imposing the rules of the mainstream society.

I began seeing Zeke twice per week; within a month, he had de-cided to make some major changes. I had already convinced him to reduce the risk of being caught stealing drugs at work by reestablish-ing his old contact or by limiting himself to the opium that he grew on his own. When he decided that it was best not to find a new dealer, and when the opium was not really strong enough to hold him, a detoxification program was necessary. To my surprise, he agreed. Because of his work, Zeke refused to participate in any struc-tured program. In consultation with a private physician, an expert in this area, Zeke completed a 2-week detoxification from narcotics at home, using prescribed benzodiazepines (diazepam) and pot. He had several friends stay with him for support, but he refused to come in to therapy until he was feeling better. I did convince him to have phone contact with me a few times during the detox. He seemed amazed that I would want to talk with him while he was sick.

With the detoxification complete, Zeke was ready to examine the reasons for his use and to deal with his life in general. I began to notice several themes in our sessions. A combination of his irritability (that predated his withdrawal from narcotics), and a lack of real pleasure

("My life is fine; why am I so bored and dissatisfied?") led me to refer him for a fuller assessment. Despite the fact that long-term marijuana use can cause this constellation of symptoms, he had a sad, painful air to him that led me to guess that he was suffering from a masked depression, a subtype that is most typical of men in our society. The consulting psychiatrist agreed, and Zeke began taking Zoloft, with amazing results. Within a month, he was smiling and joking; he felt motivated to work on intimacy issues in therapy, considered looking for different work, and was ready to deal with his drug problems.

Despite (or because of) his awareness that drugs impaired his willingness to go out into the world of people, Zeke was unsure how much he wanted to change. He was glad to be off the narcotics, but mostly because of the legal dangers. He claimed that marijuana was a poor substitute, but he continued to use it. I convinced him to schedule his pot smoking rather than just use it when he felt like it. He did manage to moderate his use of marijuana and abstain from alcohol for long periods of time, with occasional slips into more heavy use, and a few episodes of opium use.

After the first 8 months, Zeke's treatment focused increasingly on his social isolation and feelings of profound sadness and loneliness, dating from his childhood. He felt now, as he had then, that while people could care about him, no one could really be of much use when he really needed advice or help. I brought our growing relationship to his attention and pushed him to struggle with a new and different reality, that someone might actually both care about him and be of some help to him. He began to experience our relationship as different from his expectations, but only when he was in the room with me. His attachment was not yet strong enough to hold onto my image when we were not together. I increased his sessions to three times per week, and the issue of dependability became central. With the additional contact, Zeke was able to understand the profound intimate relationship that he had developed with his drugs over the years and why living without them felt intolerable: With drugs, he could allow himself to experience a need and fulfill it, with a certainty that one cannot expect from people. Unlike many other people with serious drug problems, he was able to function normally in the world, safe in the nurturing narcotic haze. Zeke continues to work on letting go of the certainty of drugs in favor of the uncertain, but more satisfying, world of people.

## BETWEEN TWO WORLDS:
## THE CASE OF BHATI

It is not uncommon for a psychotherapist to begin treatment with the idea that drug use is not an issue for a patient. This does not necessarily mean that the person is hiding his use, but he may indicate that the use is not a problem, or he may not know that it is. This presentation is typical of people in the precontemplation stage of change.

Bhati was 20 years old but appeared no more than 16. He and his family had emigrated from Thailand more than 3 years earlier but had been living in the Midwest. Bhati had recently moved to California to attend school, and he had a difficult time adjusting to his new life as a student in a large urban area. He was referred to me after a nurse at the university student health center became concerned that he was losing weight and appeared depressed.

Bhati did not appear depressed to me so much as shy and perhaps tired. I asked him if he was getting enough sleep, and he giggled and had a slightly guilty look. I commented that young men often try to do many things at once and sometimes forget to sleep. This statement seemed to indicate to him that I was used to whatever his habits might be, and he was then quite open about what had brought him to "the doctor."

He and his family (two sisters, two brothers, and parents) had moved to the United States after spending years in waiting camps or with relatives in Thailand. He remembered being bored and hungry at that time, but never frightened. After relocating, his family lived in a rural area in the Midwest and worked on local farms and in stores. Bhati finished high school, won a scholarship to a prestigious university, and so became the first of his family to go to college. He was working as well as attending school full time, and he was proud to be able to send money home to his family.

I spent several sessions with Bhati, following his lead in the conversation. I had learned from previous experience that people from Thailand are often superficially friendly to strangers, which does not necessarily indicate that they are giving you permission to broach more personal topics. In addition, my status as a professional was likely to engender feelings in him of both respect and a suspicion that I would pass judgment on his behavior. Some of my (and his) concerns about our relating to each other had to do with cultural differences; others, for him, seemed to be the typical concerns and defenses of a young man talking with a mature woman. As he talked about his current life, I commented on the naturalness of his concerns: "After all, you are a young man with hopes and dreams, in a new country, learning the language and customs." After several introductory sessions, I guessed correctly that he was feeling lonely for companionship and gently inquired about "romance." Bhati hesitantly told me that while he had several girlfriends at home, since he had been in America, "no girl touches me."

It was not until Bhati and I had been meeting for several months and focusing on his loneliness that I felt comfortable making some pointed inquiries about his life. It took very little persuasion to get him to disclose that he was using hallucinogens and alcohol in large quantities on the weekends. At first, he reported this with a self-righteousness typical of many men who feel stressed out by work. He had "earned" his binges and saw no problem with them. I allowed that he must, indeed, have earned the right to pleasure and relaxation given how hard he worked during the week. With this affirmation of his reality, he described in detail his current and past substance use history, which did not sound to me like an innocuous program of tension relief.

Bhati had been drinking alcohol since he was 14 years old, usually on the weekends; at times of great stress, he would drink during the week as well. All of his friends and family members drank alcoholic beverages, so he saw no problems with this. He drank only moderately, usually three or four beers at time. After coming to California, however, he had found it difficult to purchase alcohol, since he was not old enough and looked even younger than his age. His pattern of use had changed dramatically. He now drank only on weekends and had a friend buy a case of beer for him, which he drank over a 24-hour period. He also began smoking marijuana and taking psychedelics such as LSD along with the alcohol. Bhati was now clearly using drugs to obliterate any sense of reality. The types and quantities could not be viewed as merely "recreational" use, even though he typically used only 1 or 2 days each week. In addition, the pattern did not conform to any particular Asian subgroup of which I was aware.

Unfortunately, there are not many studies that differentiate among Asian people from different countries (Varma & Siris, 1996) in terms of risk and prevalence for alcohol and drug problems. Education, family coherence, and language and job skills are, in general, protective factors for immigrant Asian groups. Yee and Thu (1987) found that among high-risk Indochinese refugees, the incidence of alcohol problems was about 45%. This study points out, however, that because so many of the refugees were single men living alone or in unrelated communal settings, the results are probably not representative of the entire ethnic community. Despite little guidance from the literature, I made a few decisions about how I would approach the treatment with Bhati and took note of his response in order to alter my stance when needed.

I decided to adopt the role of a big sister or aunt, a figure who would be seen by Bhati as having both true concern for him and being in a position of authority. It seemed that the move away from his family had exacerbated whatever adjustment problems he might have had in the Midwest. He was used to depending on his family, particularly his mother, for advice on how to live. In addition to being without friends and family, he was working many hours as well as going to school. While this schedule may have kept him from feeling too badly during the week, it certainly must have contributed to his weekend binges. His English comprehension was far superior to his spoken English, creating another barrier to social interaction.

Since Bhati kept asking me the name for his problem, I decided to give him a diagnosis of "dislocation grief"; with that, I was able to help him normalize the many thoughts, feelings, and behaviors that were troublesome to him. The combination of his youth, gender, and ethnicity made it important for me to align with his self-esteem, pride, and self-efficacy rather than pathologize his difficulties. This "dislocation grief," I said, was the normal reaction to leaving one's home and family and beginning a new life. I used the decisional balance with him to look at the excitements and the losses he was experiencing, and I stressed the importance of respecting all of his opposing feelings. Together, Bhati and I created a ritualized style of therapy in which he would arrive with a very grave expression and announce that the "grief and joy is with me." I would then encourage him to stand still and face both the grief and the joy in order to avoid further "dislocation" of his spirit. I avoided any mention of his behavior outside of the therapy room, hoping I could first create a balanced emotional life within the confines of our relationship.

Within 4 months, Bhati mentioned that he was not standing still and facing his grief and joy in his outside life. He was experiencing a dissociation that made him sufficiently uncomfortable to realize he would have to change first his drinking and drug use, then his social life. Once Bhati labeled his drug and alcohol use as a problem, I again took an active "aunt-like" role, reminding him that in order to grow up in his new country, he would have to be clearheaded and honest. Over the next few months, we talked about balancing his lifestyle to allow more freedom during the week and thus reduce his need to blow off steam on the weekends. I put him in touch with a local Asian American youth club and suggested additional tutoring in English as way of holding both cultures inside him. Bhati stopped his drug use and reduced his drinking to a few beers on weekend nights. He seemed happier and proud of his accomplishments. We parted with my promise to think of him and his promise to think of himself also.

## CONCLUSIONS

Each of these clinical cases challenges us to rethink how to approach a person with drug and alcohol problems. No therapeutic intervention is independent of the relationship that develops between clinician and client. Special attention needs to be paid to this process.

It is clear from the previous section that matching a particular patient to a particular treatment is an art. Such matching has yet to be systematically studied. The paucity of research in the area of alternative treatment approaches slows the progress of the profession and makes some clinicians wary to try a new approach. However, extensive research in the field shows that an unwillingness to discuss "taboo topics" (those that go against traditional methods of chemical dependency treatment) stalls the development of sound therapeutic strategies and theories (Chiauzzi & Liljegren, 1993). In psychotherapy, failure to offer "taboo" options to patients often increases resistance at a fragile point in the development of the therapeutic relationship. Since treatment retention has been shown to be the primary factor in positive outcome with addictions, it is essential that treatments be modified or developed with the purpose of holding the patient in treatment, and with less rigidity to a particular model. I have tried to show both the flexibility and the thoughtful construction of the therapeutic strategy that is at the heart of harm reduction psychotherapy.

# CHAPTER SIX

# *Dual- and Multidiagnosis Patients*

$M$uch controversy surrounds the issue of dual diagnosis. Both the public and private health care systems continue to struggle with the problem of attending to the needs of a drug-using population in the current climate of zero tolerance and the War on Drugs. For years, mental health professionals and chemical dependency specialists spent valuable time shuttling certain patients back and forth between the two systems of care. Mental health workers felt unprepared and/or unwilling to address issues of alcohol or drug use, while chemical dependency workers had little idea how to cope with a schizophrenic patient or someone with severe anxiety. When, in response to clinician frustration, administrative rules were developed for patients' entry and retention in treatment programs, some of these policies actually excluded many of the most needy and difficult patients from necessary treatment.

In addition, 12-Step programs' refusal in the past to allow clients to use any psychoactive medications prevented most mental health patients from entering into chemical dependency treatment. Those who entered without their medications often suffered relapses of both their psychiatric and drug problems. Clinicians have dubbed these patients "double trouble," a pejorative term that speaks to the continuing attitude in the field that dual-diagnosis patients are the most difficult to treat. This is certainly true in many cases. However, if one takes the view that *all* serious addictions are accompanied by significant emotional problems, then it is easier to realize that many clients will present as dually diagnosed.

## COMORBIDITY

Recent research shows that there are a significant number of dual-diagnosis patients in the general population, as well as a majority of persons in patient populations. The results of the 1990 Epidemiologic Catchment Area Study (Regier et al., 1990) indicate that of those people in the general population with a mental disorder, 29% will also have an alcohol or drug disorder at some point in their lives. When people with alcohol disorders were screened, 37% had a mental disorder; while those persons with a drug disorder were not only seven times more likely to have an alcohol disorder, but also 53% had a mental disorder. These comorbidity percentages increase dramatically in patient samples, showing that up to 78% of people in treatment for a drug or alcohol disorder also have a mental disorder.

It is clear from the research that psychiatric disorders are prevalent in the substance-abusing population (Ries, 1994). One thing that is not obvious in this research, however, is that some of these disorders are substance induced and do not exist independently of the alcohol or drug use. Estimates of alcohol-induced depression, for example, suggest that as many as 65% of patients admitted for alcohol treatment who are depressed at the time of intake will not be depressed after 3 weeks. (Some clinicians suggest that dysthymic disorder, however, does not usually remit with abstinence, but since only major depression is listed, the statistics may be misleading.) Conventional wisdom states that you cannot reliably differentiate between psychiatric (functional) disorders and drug-induced (organic) disorders for days, if not weeks, after acute or chronic intoxication. Several researchers assert, however, that it is possible to differentiate between substance-induced and independent depressive episodes by using standard depression inventories (Shukit, 1989). The issue is not merely academic. Untreated major depression is a significant cause of relapse into active alcoholism (Hasin et al., 1996), and untreated bipolar disorder makes abstinence from stimulants almost impossible.

In general, history is often the only reliable way to make differential decisions. Even then, often the best one can do is determine what is *not* the problem! Very often, the current symptoms reflect only a short-term change in the course of a long-term disorder. There are some shortcuts and hints to assist the clinician in assessing the relative influence of each disorder in a multidisordered patient. The pharmacology of certain drugs allows us either to rule out or raise our index of suspicion when we see certain symptoms. See Appendix A for pharmacology information.

## DIFFERENTIAL DIAGNOSIS BY TYPE OF DRUG

The type of substance used will dictate critical features of the syndrome observed. Symptoms vary depending on withdrawal or acute intoxication. This section presents a list of drugs and the psychiatric conditions that may mimic or be caused by the drug's effects.

### Stimulants

Acute intoxication may resemble various agitated states or paranoid psychosis. In addition, chronic use of stimulants can induce syndromes that are difficult to distinguish from mania or schizophrenia. Nicotine in ordinary doses does not cause symptoms that mimic any psychological disorder, but it may contribute to underlying agitation.

Withdrawal can mimic agitated depression with severe suicidal ideation, depending on amount and duration of substance use. With stimulant use, unlike major depression, the suicidal ideation often clears within 48 hours. Withdrawal from nicotine may cause significant agitation, anxiety, and insomnia but does not generally fit the profile of any major mental disorder.

### Sedatives

Acute intoxication may result in violent behavior, seriously impaired judgment, and poor motor skills. If a patient is depressed while using, suicidality is increased. Alcohol may also cause such extreme symptoms but usually only in very high doses.

Withdrawal can be severe, with prominent anxiety, rebound insomnia, seizures, psychosis, and death. It generally takes at least 10–14 days to differentiate between functional and withdrawal psychosis. It may take 2–3 weeks for depression to subside. See Appendix A for a more detailed description of the signs of, and treatment for, alcohol withdrawal.

## Hallucinogens

Acute intoxication resembles brief psychosis and other psychotic-like alterations in perception and thought. Panic attacks may occur.

There is no known withdrawal syndrome for these drugs.

## Opiates

Acute intoxication causes symptoms that range from lethargy to somnolence that may be severe enough to mimic organic brain disorders. If significant depression is present, it usually represents a psychiatric problem because, paradoxically, narcotic drugs do not tend to cause depression even with chronic use. Major depressive disorder is relatively common as a comorbid condition, though, and can be treated successfully with medications even in opiate-dependent people (Nunes, Quitkin, Donovan, & Deliyannides, 1998).

Withdrawal results in a characteristic flu-like syndrome. Anxiety is prominent and will remit with medical detoxification or with time. In general, no psychiatric syndromes mimic this process. The most common differential diagnosis is with organic syndromes, however. Falls and blows to the head may result in brain trauma. Note problems with attention, concentration, memory, and emotional lability; opioids do not generally cause these cognitive problems in either intoxication or withdrawal phases.

## Miscellaneous Substances
## (Solvents, Anticholinergics)

These drugs often directly cause organic brain syndromes. Differential diagnosis must include laboratory testing, pharmacological challenges, and time. Profound mental status changes are seen (attention problems, alterations in level of consciousness, motor incoordination).

## DIFFERENTIAL DIAGNOSIS BY PSYCHIATRIC DISORDER

Another way of ordering one's thoughts is by thinking of psychiatric syndromes first. The major syndromes for differential diagnosis are affective disorders, anxiety disorders, psychotic disorders, and organic brain syndromes.

### Depression

Depression is very common among substance abusers. During withdrawal, it can be caused by either stimulants or sedatives and usually resolves within 2–3 weeks. Some depression may persist for a few months. Persons who are suicidal should be considered for standard psychiatric treatment (medications and therapy), as should anyone with a clear history of depressive episodes while clean and sober.

### Mania

Mania can be induced by stimulants and may be an exacerbation of bipolar disorder or an organic mania. There is no good way to tell the difference except by history. If possible, the person should be assessed when drug free.

### Anxiety

Anxiety may be increased or decreased by drugs and alcohol. Panic attacks can be induced by either acute cocaine ingestion or opioid withdrawal. This is not the same as a panic disorder, which is rare in substance abusers. In general, alcohol temporarily helps persons with social phobias but not those with panic disorder.

### Psychosis

Schizophrenia is often misdiagnosed in stimulant abusers. Toxicology results are essential, as is a longitudinal assessment while the patient is drug free. However, even if the drug panel is positive for stimulants, it is impossible to know if the stimulants caused the psychosis. On the other hand, a negative drug panel is a good indication that the psychosis is part of a psychiatric disorder or other organic condition. Persons with schizophrenia are highly sensitive to most drugs and will exhibit substantial symptoms with even small amounts of drug. Opioid and alcohol use may reduce psychotic symptoms temporarily, whereas withdrawal will make them worse. Cocaine has been shown to decrease negative symptoms (social withdrawal, anhedonia, cognitive slowing), while causing more of the positive symptoms (hallucinations, delusions, agitation) typical in a frank psychotic episode (Dixon, Haas, & Weiden, 1990).

### Substance-Induced Disorders
### (Organic Brain Syndromes)

This group of disorders is significantly worsened and may be precipitated by any kind of drug use. For example, Wernicke's syndrome is a dementia caused by alcohol, and AIDS-induced encephalopathy is dramatically increased with stimulant use. Geriatric patients using sedatives are at risk of increasing symptoms, especially confusion. All types of dementia are made worse by the use of drugs. Benzodiazepines can cause confusion or a paradoxical agitation, as can alcohol. It is essential to get a thorough neurological workup if any of these conditions are suspected. Many can be treated effectively, and some leave lasting brain damage if not treated quickly.

## A HIERARCHY OF NEEDS
## WITH DUAL-DIAGNOSIS PATIENTS

There is no easy way to assess the relative impact of drugs on mental conditions. The information in this section should be used as a guide to clinical interviewing. Obviously, the more one knows about drug pharmacology and the natural course of mental disorders, the better chance one has of correctly putting the pieces together. The best test is time and a good therapeutic relationship with the patient. It has been shown that dual-diagnosis patients in a supportive, nonpunitive atmosphere are quite honest about their drug-taking activities

(Weiss, Najavits, Greenfield, & Soto, 1998). It is possible to begin treatment even without a firm diagnosis, however. One can use the following hierarchy of needs to guide the initial phases of treatment. This hierarchy in turn can be used as a treatment protocol, with tasks assigned to various staff in multidisciplinary settings. For example, the following hierarchy can be used for a person presenting in crisis at an acute facility (psychiatric or medical):

Develop rapport.
Stabilize dangerous symptoms or behaviors.
Assess state of intoxication, withdrawal, or acute decompensation.
Treat acute medical problems (includes refilling prescriptions).
Provide for food, shelter, and clothing.
Develop and implement plans for children or dependent adults under the patient's care.
Suggest ongoing treatments or contacts to the patient.
Inform the patient about possible links between his or her mental distress and drugs he or she may have used.
Suggest immediate interventions (abstinence, reduction of use, medications, contact with others, environmental changes, inpatient treatment).
Schedule a follow-up visit for within 3 days.

## MEDICATION STRATEGIES
## FOR DUAL-DIAGNOSIS PATIENTS

The area of psychotropic medications for dual-diagnosis patients is just being developed. There are many biases about what drugs should or should not be used with people who have addictive problems. Often, a drug with abuse potential will not be given because of a patient's *previous* drug problems, rather than because of any current abuse. While it is understandable to be cautious in prescribing psychotropic medications, it is not acceptable to withhold effective treatment *only* because of the potential harm of a patient's return to drug abuse. With treatment and education provided by both the therapist and prescribing physician, the patient is often able to follow medication guidelines and derive benefit from the treatment.

The first concerns that are usually discussed by the treatment team include decisions about the use of medications to reduce the symptoms of withdrawal. There is little disagreement at this point about the benefit of palliative treatment to reduce the stress, both physical and psychological, of withdrawal states. A difficult withdrawal is *not* a disincentive to return to drug use; rather, it sometimes delays a return to drug treatment once the person has relapsed. The word on the street is that withdrawal is horrible. If we can change that perception by the liberal use of medications, perhaps more people will enter treatment. There are many good references to guide medical detoxification (e.g., Kosten & McCance, 1996; Substance Abuse and Mental Health Services Administration, 1995).

The next decision is whether to use some type of psychotropic medication, such as an antidepressant, early in treatment or to wait a while. The question "What is a while?" is very difficult to answer. Obviously, one would offer antipsychotics or sometimes benzodiazepines (antianxiety medications) to a person whether or not the psychosis was caused by drugs, since the medication helps reduce agitation quickly. It is more difficult to decide when to begin medications for other types of symptoms. A good rule of thumb is that in the absence of clear historical diagnosis, only palliative measures should be given, and only in the lowest dose possible. An exception should be made for depression in some people. Now that it is clear that antidepressants do work for many people with dysthymic disorder, there is no reason to withhold these drugs from people who have shown clear, early-onset dysthymia. Many women fall into this category, as do some patients with a history of physical trauma. In addition, depression in opiate-dependent persons can be successfully treated with antidepressants, but this treatment may have no effect on their substance use (Nunes et al., 1998).

Treating sleep disorders in the newly abstinent patient is another complex issue. Loss of sleep increases anxiety and reduces good judgment. It is imperative to attempt quickly the restoration of as normal a sleep pattern as possible. While medications for this purpose have both their own addictive potential and the potential to cause other side effects, they must sometimes be used for a few days or weeks. Nonmedical interventions such as massage, acupuncture, herbal remedies, and instruction in sleep hygiene may help the patient.

One of the most controversial decisions is whether to offer psychiatric medications to a patient who is not abstinent. These decisions, like other medication decisions, may be recommended by any member of the treatment team, but it is ultimately the attitude of the physician that determines the outcome of treatment suggestions. An increasing body of clinical experience advocates the use of medications with actively using patients (in fact, medications have been used extensively, if unknowingly, with patients who present with psychiatric but not drug problems). But without empirically based guidelines, the prescribing practices of physicians may be restrained by their own limited experience. For example, many physicians will prescribe antipsychotics but not antidepressants under the mistaken belief that antidepressants will not work as long as a person is using, particularly if he or she is using alcohol. Other physicians are concerned with the toxicity that results when medications are combined with alcohol. While some antidepressants clearly react negatively with alcohol, others, particularly the selective serotonin reuptake inhibitors (SSRIs) do not have a predictable negative interaction. Antidepressant medications, particularly the monoamine oxidase inhibitors (MAOIs) and the tricyclic antidepressants (TCAs) do interact negatively with stimulant drugs. Even if a physician will prescribe medications such as antianxiety medications to a patient abusing alcohol, she may not prescribe an adequate dose, unaware that this person will *naturally* need increased doses for effective symptom management (Stimmel, 1997).

In terms of prescribing any particular medication to a person who may be or is actively using, there are some other considerations: Does the medication cause physiological dependence? Does the medication have street value, so that the patient might be tempted to sell it rather than take it? And, importantly, does the medication interact negatively with the person's drug of choice? This is important in the case of relapse. For instance, it would be unwise to prescribe a tricyclic antidepressant, which has potential cardiac effects, to a person with an unstable history of stimulant abuse, since stimulants often exacerbate underlying cardiac problems. In a different situation, though, it would be possible to prescribe the antidepressant Wellbutrin to a person with a history of alcohol abuse, because the two drugs do not tend to interact negatively. Obviously, the physician making the decisions should have as much training as possible in both psychopharmacology and the pharmacology of drugs of abuse in order to make effective choices. Finally, many patients will have concurrent medical illness such as HIV infection, asthma, diabetes, and so forth. It is important to determine whether a given drug is likely to cause, exacerbate, or mask symptoms of an existing medical problem. Guidance can be found in the literature, especially regarding HIV infection and substance use (see, e.g., Zweben & Denning, 1998).

The most important factor in decision making is rapport between the patient and the treatment team. Honest communication and the willingness to experiment with different medications are necessary in order to provide the most effective, and the safest, medication treatment.

## MULTIDIAGNOSIS PATIENTS:
## THE CASE OF STEVE[1]

This section explores the case of a man with a serious drug abuse problem and a severe psychiatric disorder. As if these problems were not enough for him (and me) to deal with, another disorder exaggerated and confused the clinical picture—HIV disease. The HIV epidemic presented clinicians with a frightening disease in a group of patients in the San Francisco Bay area, who were predominantly gay men. The horror of the early years of the epidemic, when one knew neither how the disease was transmitted nor how to treat it, demanded a courageous response. Professionals and the public at large responded (as a result of the insistence of the patients) by developing not only new medical treatments, but also new paradigms to provide a holistic approach to patients who brought with them other problems in addition to HIV.

### Presenting Problem

Steve, a 32-year-old white, gay male, had been seen several times for an intake appointment at a mental health clinic located in a primary

---

[1]This case is adapted from Denning (1998). Copyright 1998 by John Wiley & Sons, Inc. Adapted by permission.

care public health clinic serving HIV patients. Each time he called, he was seen by a therapist for an assessment and given a follow-up appointment that he failed to keep. At these times, he was usually in a crisis related to a failed job or relationship and had several disturbing symptoms. He appeared pressured and disorganized, yet he was seductively engaging. He seemed to welcome attention and eagerly agreed to follow-up sessions, yet he never returned and left no phone number for contact. After he called for the fourth time in as many years, I decided to see him and attempt to draw him into psychotherapy. Steve was in crisis again, and it was difficult to get him to discuss his previous clinic contacts. He did not recall ever having been seen by a psychotherapist, but he knew that he was a patient on the medical side of the clinic and was able to give the name of his physician and describe the treatment he was receiving for HIV infection. I asked the physician to step in and introduce me to her patient. This formal introduction seemed to act as a bridge, and Steve willingly agreed to work with me as his doctor's "assistant."

Over the next 2 hours, I focused on building rapport with Steve, hoping to instill in him a recognition of me as a potentially stable figure in his treatment. I instinctively avoided a formal symptom- and history-based interview, allowing him instead to tell his story as he wanted. He returned the next day to continue the evaluation process. He talked about his numerous jobs as a salesperson in a gay bookstore and, most recently, as an attendant at a local gay men's sex club. He had attended college, but he was unclear what he studied or whether he graduated. Other details of his history held no interest for him. The results of this evaluation were muddled and inconclusive.

Steve had been HIV-positive for approximately 6 years, with a current $T$-cell count that was dangerously low (75). He was essentially asymptomatic except for one occurrence of oral thrush and various, but vague, skin complaints. He was mildly euphoric and tangential, and his speech was somewhat pressured, but he responded well to structure in the interview. He complained of poor short-term memory and concentration, even though formal testing showed him to be unimpaired. He showed no evidence of psychotic thinking despite the paranoid flavor to some of his comments.

Steve's chief complaint was that he was experiencing increasing depression and dissatisfaction with his "lifestyle," which he described as "partying" and trying to make friends, who always let him down. He viewed many of these friends as trying to take advantage of his "good looks and trusting self." Further interviews revealed that he had a long history of unstable relationships, dramatic shifts in affect from happy to irritable, and dysphoria that was reactive rather than stable. He readily admitted to substance abuse, unsafe sex, and other impulsive actions that showed poor judgment. His psychiatric symptoms predated his use of drugs; thus, he met the full criteria for borderline personality disorder, with significant histrionic and narcissistic traits.

A substance-use history readily revealed a 10-year history of polysubstance abuse, including speed, cannabis, alcohol, and often "whatever was going around." He claimed to have no particular drug of choice and was unable to state exactly how much and how often he was indulging at that time. Although Steve was not defensive about his use, he expressed little motivation to change any of it. Instead, he redirected the conversation to vague complaints about his life and problems finding friends and a job. He gave many examples of his sexual prowess and claimed many jealous bosses fired him out of envy because of attention paid to him by customers at the sex clubs. He expressed some interest in 12-Step groups but would make no commitment to attend.

While clearly neither intoxicated nor psychotic at the time of intake, Steve did present with a kind of cognitive muddling and an inability to focus his thoughts for any length of time. When he expressed concern about becoming demented, I scheduled him for neuropsychological testing, both as a diagnostic tool and to emphasize to him that I wanted to be of assistance. His medical doctor eagerly cooperated by providing consultations and access to the medical records, as she was equally puzzled about his mental status. She found him charming and engaging but stated that he was often noncompliant with medical treatment recommendations, including the proper use of an antiviral medications and prophylactic treatments.

I was unable to get much psychosocial history from Steve either at intake or throughout the course of the treatment. He was born and raised in the South and apparently had at least two siblings. He referred to his father as either "fine" or "very strict and domineering." Steve made no reference to his mother except to say that he loved her. He had had no contact with his parents for many years, and they were unaware of his HIV status. I found it highly unusual to have a patient with so little interest in talking about his childhood or family. Apparently, Steve was so preoccupied with his HIV illness and his own psychological condition that his family and personal history paled in importance.

## Case Formulation:
### Treatment without Benefit of a Clear Diagnosis

Because of the severe nature of Steve's problems, it would be important for him to have regular therapy appointments. His prior failures to return for follow-up mental health treatment, even though he was responsible about medical visits, presented both a dilemma and a solution. I told Steve that he had a regular appointment to see me immediately after his appointment with either the doctor or nurse on site. Because his current HIV status did not require this intensity of medical intervention, these contacts lasted only several minutes each week. Steve came to his psychotherapy appointments regularly with this arrangement. It was clear that treatment would have to be paced to Steve's concerns or he would stop coming, as he had done in the past. I decided that the benefits of psychotherapy and regular contact were worth the risk of allowing the substance use to continue in the short run; thus, I decided to integrate substance abuse treatment into his regular psychotherapy and to adopt a harm reduction stance.

Routine blood tests were expanded to include drug toxicology tests as well. I talked with Steve about why I thought these tests were important, using his own concerns ("Am I going crazy? Am I getting HIV dementia?") as the main reason for conducting these tests, and also letting him know that I thought his ability to give accurate information about his drug use was impaired. Careful not to suggest that I thought he might be hiding or lying about his drug use, I joined with him in his attempts to be honest about his use of substances. I educated him about the symptoms that he was experiencing and the possibility that these symptoms could be caused by the drugs he was using rather than by HIV infection. For example, I cautioned him that his anxiety could possibly be exacerbated by any use of speed or cocaine, and that cognitive "muddles" might be caused by smoking marijuana. This cooperative allegiance allowed us to form an "investigative team." Together, we would look for the causes of his symptoms and his problems, and decide on a course of treatment. A re-constructed interaction clarifies this type of working style:

STEVE: I don't feel right today, but I came anyway.

PATT: I'm glad to see you, but what doesn't feel right?

STEVE: Last night started out okay, but my stupid boss couldn't stand all the attention I was getting. This rash is strange but my doctor says she can't do anything else for it.

PATT: I can't tell for sure, Steve. Are you feeling a bit frustrated with people?

STEVE: I'm not an angry person. I just don't feel right.

PATT: Well, Steve, you have a lot going on and it must be kind of confusing to figure out exactly what feels bad, huh?

STEVE: (*laughs*) You got that right, sweetheart. I'm one bitchy queen today. Got a cure for that?

PATT: Oh, sure, ask me for the impossible! (*Both of us laugh.*) But seriously, what could be causing you to be so out of sorts today? Did you drink or use any drugs yesterday?

STEVE: I'm not taking that new medicine anymore because it gives me stomach problems.

PATT: Is that the stuff for your fungal infection? You know, it some-times can also cause fatigue. Were you feeling tired, too, and didn't like that?

STEVE: I don't like any of it. The speed makes me feel better than all the medicine I've got.

PATT: Man, what a bind you're in. The stuff that's supposed to be the good medicine makes you feel sick, and the stuff that's sup-posed to be bad for you feels good. What happened to fair, huh?

STEVE: You got that right. None of it makes sense. I just don't feel good and there's nothing anyone can do.

PATT: You know, the last time you had a medicine change this hap-pened. You got some early side effects and used speed to clear them up. How about this time if you stop the medicine and see your doctor for a different kind? In the meantime, why don't you stay away from the speed for a few days until you know for sure what's going on?

STEVE: Yeah, you know, sometimes speed makes me feel funny, too. Maybe I should just take one drug at a time.

I was not sure if this agreed-upon solution would work, but it would not hurt, it might help, and, most importantly, Steve and I strengthened our bond and commitment to work together to help him in the face of his deteriorating health and pessimism.

It was an ongoing challenge to establish a diagnosis and treatment plan given the possible overlap of conditions and symptoms. Together, Steve and I, along with his physician and case manager, examined his particular complaints, the lab results, and his "objective" symptoms. I developed a formal inquiry to sort and integrate all the conflicting clinical data from these different sources. This inquiry took the form of a series of questions that were key to understanding this patient. The answers to these questions sometimes changed over time, necessitating rapid shifts in interventions.

Key Questions:

1. To what extent was his HIV infection causing his cognitive symptoms?
2. How did his use of illicit substances interact with his mental status and his medical condition?
3. How could I develop a treatment team that could work with him consistently and not get caught up in differences of opinion regarding diagnosis and appropriate treatment?
4. What might I predict about his emotional state and needs as his HIV disease worsened?
5. How might I foster a firm attachment with Steve despite his history of episodic and interrupted recourse to treatment?

## Course of Treatment

Because so many of his symptoms could be associated with any of the various drugs he was using, the therapy focused on addressing

Steve's substance abuse problems, using a harm reduction approach. I attempted to link different drugs with the symptoms he disliked in order to increase his motivation for change. His increasing paranoia was distressing to him, and he was able to notice that it got worse when he smoked pot. He decided to smoke only when he was feeling "strong." As he became more fatigued, we set up experiments in which he would use speed one evening and call me the next day to report on his level of fatigue. Then, he would abstain from speed, again calling me the next day. He quickly realized that speed use gave him only a temporary respite from fatigue and often made him feel worse the next day. Over time, these insights resulted in consistent behavioral change. At first, though, Steve would focus of this kind of work for a while but always become tangential, and the session would end with no clear plan for change.

After the results of the neuropsychological testing showed no clear evidence of dementia, Steve became more active in his treatment, disclosing feelings, behaviors, and thoughts that were disturbing to him, and asking whether a certain drug that he had taken that day could be the culprit. I gave him honest information and never overstated the possible connections or dangers. It is imperative when working with drug users to avoid the temptation to increase motivation through scare tactics. To the surprise of everyone, after only 5 months of weekly treatment, most of Steve's toxicology screenings came back negative for any illegal substance and often for alcohol as well. When asked about this, Steve admitted that he was not using "much at all" anymore because everything was beginning to make him feel paranoid.

Steve seemed unconcerned with my praise for his apparent progress, which indicated to me a lack of attachment that could jeopardize his treatment. He had no stable friends or other support group. I was concerned that his inability to form close connections was rooted in an internal alienated self (Walant, 1995) that would become more fragile as he became sicker. I offered to see him twice per week and, to my surprise, he gladly accepted.

Over the course of the next 6 months, Steve began to complain more about cognitive symptoms suggestive of early HIV dementia. At this time, the results of repeated neuropsychological testing were equivocal, and he claimed to be using no drugs at all. Instead, he was taking large doses of vitamins and herbal remedies. One winter day, he was rescued from a cold water lake where he had been swimming naked for about 1 hour. When pulled out of the cold water, his body temperature was 103 degrees Fahrenheit, and he explained that the ducks had invited him to join them. He was hospitalized and diagnosed with toxoplasmosis, a brain parasite common among HIV patients. Treatment was successful, and later magnetic resonance imaging (MRI) showed few residual lesions.

Steve became increasingly depressed and frightened about his progressing illness. He stopped socializing at all and reported no obviously self-destructive impulsive behaviors. While he could sometimes talk openly about his fear of pain and death, he did not follow through on any referrals for support groups or other potential resources. He remained drug free but began using large doses of herbal remedies, including some that contained the stimulant ephedrine. While this drug is known to cause stimulation and sometimes heart palpitations, it was unknown at the time whether it mimicked the effects of stimulant abuse, that is, paranoia and other psychotic processes. He finally accepted placement at a residential facility, where he could receive case management services. His stay was complicated by increasing paranoia about other residents as well as his haughty and critical attitude toward them. A low dose of the antipsychotic medication Mellaril was prescribed, but Steve complained of feeling drugged and would not take it regularly. He similarly refused to take antidepressant medication.

His medical doctor became frustrated with his lack of treatment compliance and his growing hostility toward her when she confronted him. Steve was transferred to another physician on site for whom he had expressed admiration. This decision was made in a joint treatment team meeting, where I facilitated the uncomfortable discussion between the devalued physician and the new, beloved one. An explanation of the rapid shifts in allegiance, trust, and cooperation that are typical of patients with borderline character structure helped ease hurt feelings and allow Steve to continue to receive care at the same facility.

Treatment continued for another 6 months, with no apparent deterioration, but with two more episodes of acute toxoplasmosis. Steve admitted to not taking his medicine regularly, again, because of paranoia. Despite his mental status, he came regularly to most appointments and maintained a working relationship with me. He was evidencing clear dependency needs at this time and was allowed phone contact as needed. Steve was unable to deal directly with his fears of dying but became more seductive and clinging, both with me and other staff at the clinic. The seductiveness consisted only of winks and coy grins, so I made no attempt to confront him about his behavior, seeing it instead as his way of both establishing and acknowledging a connection between us.

## Outcome and Prognosis

Steve continued to show improvement by maintaining stable housing, refraining from using any drugs or vitamin supplements, and coming regularly to treatment despite medical deterioration and overwhelming fears of death that he could not discuss. He would talk to me about the good times in his life as if reminiscing with an old friend. His initial distance and guarded manner evolved into a warm and open relationship with me. I helped him win a retroactive Social Security disability case that allowed him to move into his own apartment, with support care paid for by this monetary award. He usually did not appear ill but complained of feeling weak and sick all the time. He often asked my advice about a situation but would later forget that we had talked about it.

Steve called me on a Saturday evening prior to my 3-week vacation to say that he was not feeling well and was going to go to the hospital. Upon my return, I learned that he had died the day following his call to me.

## Clinical Issues

Steve was given freedom to exhibit the problem behaviors that were the reason for his seeking treatment. The fact that he had presented numerous times without follow-up made it imperative to establish contact with him that was not only nonthreatening but also designed to allow for his disorganization. It only took a brief review of his treatment history to realize that demanding immediate adherence to scheduling and abstinence from drugs would result in yet another treatment failure. His difficulty with attachment, his suspiciousness, and his growing fears about dying demanded a creative approach. Without a clear differential diagnosis, however, treatment planning became a delicate process, with much fine-tuning along the way.

Steve is typical of a growing number of patients seen in community health services (Group for the Advancement of Psychiatry, 1987). These patients are difficult to engage and retain in treatment due to disrupted mental status, drug use, and physical limitations. They also create intense emotional reactions in staff groups, causing disagreements that, unfortunately, often reduce the general quality of patient care.

Success in this case was the result of close attention to several clinical issues and the adoption of a health promotion/harm reduction stance toward Steve's problems:

1. *Willingness to experiment with engagement strategies that are flexible.* Too often, clinicians are afraid to make special arrangements with patients for fear of overstepping some arbitrarily drawn clinical boundary. Multiproblem patients require interventions that are tailored to their specific character and problems. In short, Steve was allowed to be special.

2. *Willingness to work on issues that are of stated importance to the patient rather than preconceived clinician goals.* Steve kept coming back to treatment despite being unable to articulate his needs and being dissatisfied numerous times. I had to assume that if I allowed him to lead the way, his agenda would become clearer, and together, we could formulate a plan to satisfy his needs.

3. *Willingness to act as liaison and case manager.* With multiproblem people like Steve, the traditional therapeutic stance of working within a set frame of appointment hours, for example, has to be replaced by a more flexible definition of the therapeutic relationship. Frustration of Steve's emerging dependency needs would have created a rupture in a fragile alliance. Working with him on "nontherapy" issues such as housing and scheduling increased the scope of the relationship and allowed him to develop an attachment to me via many psychological routes.

4. *Willingness to work without a diagnosis.* The difficulty in formulating a specific diagnosis, particularly when there are both organic and psychiatric symptoms, requires constant reassessment, abrupt changes in the treatment plan, and a general spirit of courage and risk taking on the part of clinicians. As the HIV epidemic grew,

our knowledge base grew as well. Members of our multidisciplinary team became more comfortable conducting treatment with only a partial knowledge of the underlying cause of a particular problem or symptom. Much time can be wasted arguing about a correct diagnosis, while the patient goes unserved.

5. *Willingness to "pass the baton" to the appropriate member of the treatment team as the case changes.* Keeping too firm a hold on one's patient is often as problematic as dumping a patient out of frustration. Issues of professional turf and authority must be examined, discussed, and resolved in order to ensure that the right clinician responds to emerging patient needs. It does no good for a therapist to interpret the meaning of a delusion if it is caused by a brain infection. Steve's hallucination, in which the ducks had invited him to come swim with them, may have had profound psychological meaning, but once the medical condition was treated, it disappeared from his awareness.

6. *Willingness to prescribe legitimate medications, including medications for pain, even if the person is using illicit drugs.* Medication issues are complex in patients with coexisting medical, psychiatric, and substance-use disorders, and must be closely monitored. It is important to remember that general guidelines for medications with dual-diagnosis patients will not be sophisticated enough for patients like Steve. A team of clinicians with expertise in pharmacology must be aware of drug interactions, and the entire team must examine its biases regarding palliative medications for substance-using patients. Providing clinicians with references and engaging in frank discussions yield the best patient care (Bezchlibnyk-Butler & Jeffries, 1998; Stimmel, 1997).

## SUMMARY AND CONCLUSIONS

The work with Steve highlights the principles of harm reduction and Addiction Treatment Alternatives. I immediately enlisted a group of professionals to plan care that was based on this patient's requests and felt needs. These services were offered with as few restrictions or barriers as possible (flexible appointment times, unscheduled contact). In addition, I developed an intervention plan that assumed Steve could participate in his own treatment despite the effects of polysubstance use on his mental status. And, importantly, I carefully paired Steve's description of negative emotional experiences to his use of certain drugs. I struck a balance between ignoring the drug use as a mere symptom of his underlying psychopathology and focusing on the drug use as the primary concern. This constellation of principles and interventions created a working therapeutic partnership with a man who had never before maintained a stable relationship. I believe that the results would have been very different had I used traditional chemical dependency treatment methods. Most likely, Steve would not have returned for regular care. If he had, one could envision a constant, frustrating cycle of confrontation, denial, paranoia, and treatment dropout.

This case was more complicated than many that we deal with in our general psychotherapy practices. Nonetheless, these principles and attitudes can be used with all patients. Since I have begun to use a harm reduction approach with my dual-diagnosis patients, I am astonished by the shift in the work. Resistance is replaced by cooperation, and honest communication builds a therapeutic relationship that I had struggled to establish using standard dynamic psychotherapeutic techniques.

I owe whatever wisdom I now possess to the patients who taught me that they do indeed know what they want and will allow me to help if I do not stand in their way.

# PART *III*

---

# *INTEGRATING THE NEW WITH THE OLD*

CHAPTER SEVEN

# *Harm Reduction Psychotherapy: Applications and Adjustments*

$M$ost of the previous discussions have been clinical in nature, focusing on the assessment and treatment of individuals. While I developed Addiction Treatment Alternatives (ATA) initially as a harm reduction psychotherapy model, it quickly evolved into one applicable to clinical consultation, staff training, and organizational development as well. This chapter presents two examples of applications in settings other than psychotherapy. The AIDS Housing Project is an example of an organizational development project whose goal was to combine the principles of harm reduction within the structure of an existing program as well as to offer suggestions on the development of new ones. Next is a case consultation project based on a patient within a community mental health service. I collected clinical information from several sources and presented the case to a multidisciplinary team of clinicians.

In addition to applications of a harm reduction model, there are many adjustments that need to be made to standard psychotherapy practice, as well as limitations and ethical considerations that are just now being recognized. The end of this chapter discusses some of these issues and invites the reader to think about the possibilities and dilemmas offered by harm reduction psychotherapy.

## THE AIDS HOUSING PROJECT

Early in 1998, I was invited to provide training and consultation in harm reduction to a number of agencies in San Francisco that provide housing, and associated services for people with HIV. These programs, which received funding from the federal Housing and Urban Development Department (HUD) under legislation entitled "Housing Opportunities for People with AIDS" (HOPWA), were also under the direction of the local San Francisco Department of Public Health. A conflict had arisen between federal mandates for a drug-free, zero-tolerance policy regarding drug use on the one hand, and local interest in providing housing for people who are at the greatest risk of being homeless—the poor, mentally ill, and/or substance-abusing person with AIDS—on the other. Because of different funding sources, there were various policies and program language that applied to some agencies, but not others. For example, in state-licensed agencies such as skilled nursing facilities, drug activity on site is specifically prohibited, whereas city-funded programs often had abstinence language only in program mission statements. Moreover, the Community Substance Abuse Services of the Department of Public Health had recently mandated that all treatment programs include harm reduction strategies. While the HOPWA agencies were not treatment facilities, but housing with support services, the move toward harm reduction was mandated for them as well.

The San Francisco Redevelopment Agency, with funding from a technical assistance grant to the Corporation for Supportive Housing (CSA), provided the leadership for this venture. Along with the Department of Public Health, it wanted to implement a new programmatic model but had no concept of what that would or should be. While many of the program supervisors and directors had the expertise to rework the culture of their organizations, few had the necessary understanding of harm reduction to orchestrate significant program changes in this regard. Over a period of 4 months, I worked with 12 different housing agencies, ranging from an 8-bed skilled nursing facility in a quiet residential neighborhood to a 45-bed support services facility in the heart of a drug ridden inner-city area. I met with agency directors and their supervisory staff, property managers, and frontline staff, including nursing assistants and clerks, case managers, money managers, food service workers, nurses, and social workers. In several cases, I met directly with the residents of the programs as well.

While the goal of the consultation project was to instruct agency personnel in the principles and techniques of harm reduction in order to help them work with residents still using drugs, the actual work went far beyond this simple training task. Certain funding sources put program directors under pressure to include harm reduction language in their funding proposals, program reports, and program policy statements, while simultaneously maintaining a sobriety model. In addition, most of the programs had resident intake sheets stating clearly that no drug or alcohol use would be permitted under penalty of eviction. A sticking point with this policy is that after 28 days, people enjoy tenants' rights and cannot be evicted from housing solely because they have committed an illegal act. How, then, were these programs to proceed? Many of them advertised as "clean and sober housing," and people came to live there expecting support for their sobriety. In addition, many of the programs included an array of support services offered by staff that invariably included several persons who were "in recovery" themselves. Confusion, misunderstanding, fear, and resistance existed alongside excitement about new ideas and a firm commitment on everybody's part to help the residents who counted on them.

The consultation usually developed out of needs expressed by the program director of the facility. Before meeting the entire staff, I first met with the director, and sometimes with supervisory staff as well, to review the basic concepts of harm reduction and answer questions. There were many misconceptions to clear up. During a full staff training, I remember hearing one person ask whether or not he should "do harm reduction on" a person who was continuing to use despite participating in drug treatment. Others assumed that harm reduction meant that they could not talk to a person about her drug use unless she initiated the conversation. *The biggest misconception, however, was that harm reduction and abstinence are in opposition to each other.*

Another problem that had to be addressed immediately was the tendency of people to divide into camps favoring or opposing harm reduction. I spent much time helping people understand that *one cannot be for or against harm reduction—it is what people do all the time*. I used examples from everyday life to help people realize that harm reduction, as a philosophy, allows for many different implementation strategies, abstinence being one of them. If there were refreshments offered at the meeting, I would take a piece of fruit and say that I had just implemented a harm reduction strategy for myself: I could have had a doughnut! I asked how many people had gotten a flu shot and pointed out that this, too, is a harm reduction strategy. The most important point that I made over and over again is that *there is a continuum of harm reduction strategies for every problem, and there is room for all of us to have our own beliefs and limits about which ones we use.*

In this early process, it was important to defuse any fighting that might have resulted from people's fear of change. I realized quickly that if the program was to benefit from my assistance, it would be essential to bring people along a cooperative track. I enjoyed this process immensely. The workers were clearly dedicated people who wanted to provide the best possible living situation for all of the residents and were afraid that a few problematic people would make life unbearable for them all. They were acutely aware that in any residential setting, the good of the individual might have to be sacrificed for the good of the group. They feared that implementing harm reduction in their agency would result in a tyranny of the individual.

## Developing a New Culture (Staff and Residents)

Many of the programs had been in existence for at least 1 year, and some for as long as 10 years. During this time, the program had developed a particular culture that defined expectations of each person, staff members and residents alike. Some programs had actively worked to create a sense of community within the house by having resident meetings that encouraged input and regular contact between staff and residents. While none of these agencies were considered treatment facilities (they were merely housing), most of them offered services that blurred the boundaries between treatment, case management, and housing. Despite not being treatment oriented, many of the staff had clinical degrees or drug and alcohol certificates. One such program, a 45-bed skilled nursing facility specifically designed to provide permanent housing to people with HIV, substance abuse, and psychiatric disorders, represents a good example of this mixture of services. During staff training there, as I inadvertently offered several suggestions on a particular case, one of the staff members said, "But we're not a treatment program." It amazed me that after only 3 hours with this staff, I had fallen into the dilemma that they face each day in their work: How much disruption secondary to psychiatric symptoms should they tolerate; and to what extent should they intervene to help residents overcome their problems? To do this would be a far cry from just providing permanent housing and nursing services, but not to do this meant that some of these multidiagnosed people would not be able to maintain their housing.

All of these issues represent the culture and the community sense in each setting that I entered. Whenever change is introduced into an organization, particularly an apparent about-face from the status quo, individuals must be given time to readjust and redefine their role in the organization. Without time to discuss, question, and share input, staff will have difficulty feeling that they belong to the program anymore, and may also feel that their previous work is being devalued. Some staff will embrace the changes and become active participants in the development of the new organizational culture, while others may inadvertently sabotage the efforts of those seeking change. It was important for me to present the problems, state the potential areas of disagreement, and then invite the staff to air their personal views and feelings in the spirit of honoring everybody's ideas. The intent of this type of consultation is not only to help create change, but also to ensure that those who object to it have their dissenting opinions heard and respected. Covert grumbling and passive resistance are the products of lack of respect for the difficulties inherent in making significant changes, whether personal or organizational.

## Changing Mission Statements, Rules, and Regulations

Several of the agencies were under time pressure to rewrite their program mission statements and had little idea how to go about it given that they had to please any number of funding sources. Since all of these agencies were serving people with a serious medical disorder, HIV, I helped them design a mission statement whose primary concept was health promotion. With this in mind, we were able to create a program model that encouraged abstinence from drugs and alcohol while accepting the inevitability that some residents would use. The goal was to promote healthy activities without punishing people for their drug problems by forcing them out of their homes.

## Focus on Behaviors, Not Drugs

Central to a harm reduction philosophy is the acceptance that some people will at times use drugs or alcohol even when they are attempting to remain abstinent. Others have made no commitment to themselves to be drug free. Reducing harm within a residential community when one cannot absolutely enforce a ban on drug use presented a unique challenge for these agencies. I assisted the program members, staff and residents alike, to reorient their thinking so that disruptive or disrespectful *behaviors*, rather than drug use, became the focus for rules and interventions. A resident banging on another's door at 3:00 A.M. looking for matches to light his crack pipe is a typical example of disruptive behavior, but prior to this training, the typical response was to focus on the drug use as the problem rather than the door banging. As I asked staff for specific examples of drug use and the problems it was causing in the house, we were able to translate the examples into behavioral rules of conduct for the residents. As often as possible, these rules were stated as health-promotion activities rather than prohibitions. One agency changed its curfew rule to state that it wanted people to be in the house late in the evenings to prepare for sleep, since rest is important to the maintenance of good health. No rule was set saying that residents could not stay out as late as they pleased, but if the pattern was recurrent, the staff could initiate a discussion about residents' need for sleep and encourage people to make an effort to change. If a person's drug use might contribute to the lack of sleep, that issue would also be a focus of discussion.

Not all problems can be rephrased in this way, of course. People high on drugs often are unaware of how their behavior affects other people. Generic rules and clear prohibitions may be necessary. Whenever possible, these rules should come from resident concerns as well as staff issues. One group of residents suggested two basic rules: (1) Do not knock on someone's door after 10:00 P.M., and (2) do not offer to sell drugs to another resident. Programs that have licensing requirements concerning illegal drugs on the premises will also have to set a clear rule forbidding possession, but they may not need to follow it up with punitive sanctions. When programs focus on disruptive behaviors, residents' rights to make choices about their drug use are respected, and at the same time, any harm to the community is minimized.

## The Resident Community

Harm reduction evolved as a "bottom-up" endeavor, coming from the stated needs of drug users rather than from health providers. This history helps us focus on who is really in charge of each person's life and forces us to decide if we as professionals are willing to share the power of planning and decision making with the people using the services we fund and staff. Several agencies were comfortable enough with the basic concepts of harm reduction to introduce the ideas to residents and involve them in the change process. In contrast to many practitioners' belief that psychiatric patients, let alone drug addicts, are incapable of rational input in programmatic decisions, the staff at these agencies were eager to have residents join them in changing the culture and developing a better sense of community.

In a large room, surrounded by staff and residents, I felt very much at home. Years ago, I directed a residential facility before moving to outpatient work, and found I retained an understanding of and fondness for the process of involving people in their own change while attempting to run a facility with the least amount of disruption. The residents at one agency ran the gamut from those obviously debilitated by HIV to those who, thanks to the new protease inhibitor drug cocktails, were apparently healthy. Some were articulate, others quiet, silenced at times by their own psychiatric symptoms. Several appeared to be either intoxicated or recuperating from a binge of one sort or another. After a brief introduction by the program director, I began talking about harm reduction and what it means, then asked to hear residents' concerns about people using drugs in their community.

I am not sure exactly what I expected, but the variety of responses was surprising to me and took a while to digest. During the meetings I focused on hearing residents' specific concerns, translating them into behaviors that people found disruptive, then asking for possible solutions. Typical concerns included not wanting other residents to borrow money from them, being angry when someone obviously high on speed could not sit still in the television room or changed the channel without asking, and being disturbed when wakened by someone coming in late at night. Others raised the problem of verbal altercations between residents, which seemed most likely to take place when one of the participants was intoxicated. It was surprising how much easier it was for the residents than for the staff to redirect their comments about drug use to specific problem behaviors. Clearly, whereas residents saw drugs as a problem in general, it was specific disruptive behaviors that affected them most keenly.

Interestingly, behaviors were not residents' only concern. Many voiced opinions and values that were important to them. Some asserted that everyone ought to make his or her own decisions, without pressure from others, as long as they did not take advantage of others. A few residents stated that they did not want to have to be in the same house with drug users, fearing that negative behaviors couldn't be controlled, or that their own cravings would be triggered. *This issue, feeling threatened and worried about returning to drug use if others were using, must be aggressively addressed if all residents are to feel safe and comfortable.*

I offered several intervention strategies. Since safety was the underlying concern, I suggested that staff design an intervention strategy to use with resident drugs users and communicate that plan to all the other residents. For example, one agency, as part of its mission statement, outlined the process to be followed when a person's behavior was disruptive secondary to drug use. The resident would be isolated in his or her room if necessary and a "debriefing" would occur as soon as possible. The purpose of this talk was to help the resident articulate why he or she used at that particular time and to supply the user with information about what behaviors were disruptive. This debriefing would be followed up in the weekly community meeting by a report of incidents that had occurred during the week and staff response to them. In this way, residents, while not being able to actually control someone else's drug use, could be reassured that it would not go unnoticed and that staff were actively involved in solving the problem.

Although all residents understood that their housing agreement required them to be abstinent, the general attitude of many was "Live and let live." Many of them had at times either been homeless or had lived in substandard, unstable housing and understood implicitly the threat of eviction and its disastrous consequences. Residents were generally unwilling to report drug use to staff if this resulted in someone being put out on the street. Once they understood that under the new harm reduction policy, no one would be evicted just for drug use, they began to see the possibilities for more active involvement in monitoring other resident's behavior.

Residents made it clear in these meetings that they were not entirely satisfied that staff were doing their part to control problems and they expected staff to take a primary role in protecting them from problems caused by others in the house using drugs. Residents of one program complained that staff often did not intervene in arguments or disruptive situations at all, or would wait until a situation had escalated and then tell everyone to calm down, not just the offending person. This style of general recrimination is often seen in families where the parent is frustrated and unsure how to intervene fairly, so he or she sends all the kids to their rooms, with the result that some of the kids end up feeling unjustly accused and resentful. The program director and I were glad to hear this information from the residents, and we began to make plans to address the problem. I suggested that the agency request technical assistance from the Corporation for Supportive Housing to train staff in basic skills of conflict resolution, deescalation, mediation, and so forth. One mistake supervisors often make when introducing major changes is to spend all the training time on concepts and rules, without offering specific skills training so that these rules can be implemented with confidence.

## The Staff Community

Program staff were intensely involved in the consultations and trainings. The group worked hard and cared deeply about the residents under their care. The diversity of people and opinions within the staff made it impossible to devise simplistic solutions or prematurely forge ahead with consensus about program development. We talked about the need for an ongoing dialogue about harm reduction as it affected both staff members personally and their work, and the program on a day-to-day basis. I attempted to create an atmosphere with staff that accepted individual differences and at the same time strongly challenged their usual ideas. While many staff members were already interested in harm reduction, and most were actually using the basic principles at least some of the time, the intensity of the training and the changes proved upsetting to some staff members. It was remarkable to me the number of programs and individual staff members that were already using harm reduction techniques. This usually took the form of offering residents many chances to change their drug use, active assistance in terms of referrals to treatment programs, and informal talks prior to considering eviction. The staff were obviously aware of their mission: to provide permanent housing (in most cases) to people at high risk for becoming homeless. Toward this end, they were willing to engage in a prolonged series of interventions before feeling they had to take the extreme action of eviction. Despite their dedication and pragmatic practices, all of the staff had significant concerns to be addressed and problems to be solved in order for them to participate fully in these radical organizational changes.

One of the most serious conflicts raised was about the fundamental stance of advocating abstinence as opposed to tolerating continued drug use. Staff were concerned that adopting a harm reduction model would represent condoning drug use in a population that often had already suffered serious consequences from drugs. In order to facilitate increased flexibility, I kept returning to two realities. First, people are going to do what they are going to do, despite our, and their, best intentions. Our choice is whether to continue to help them if they make choices with which we do not agree. Second, the staff's *job* is to make sure that these people do not lose their housing. While this emphasis did not satisfy everyone, it gave each person a framework for his or her ideas.

Of course many of the staff in some programs were former alcohol and drug users themselves, currently in recovery with the help of 12-Step programs. Their discomfort with harm reduction had additional dimensions that they discussed openly. Because they believed addiction to be a progressive disease, it was impossible for them to accept the fact that a person might be able to use drugs responsibly. One concern was that taking care of people's basic needs while they were actively using might actually prevent or delay their entry into treatment, making the program destructive to people by delaying or preventing them from stopping their drug use. These ideas forced me to remember a disquieting fact about harm reduction; that is, it is a relatively new paradigm, and those of us who espouse it have little idea of its limitations in application. Focusing on the obvious good that could come from it, we hardly examine the potential pitfalls, the harm that harm reduction techniques might inadvertently cause some people. In time, we will have to return to this question, as well as to particular clients with whom we work in order to assess the results of our strategies. Five years from now we may be better able to match the needs of a person with a particular intervention and make an educated guess as to whether a confrontational or supportive approach is likely to work best.

Meanwhile, other staff members in 12-Step recovery programs hinted that being around drug users, even when these people were clients rather than friends, was threatening to them. The cravings they felt were uncomfortable and scary. Because this worry was also expressed by several residents, I decided to work on the issue from the perspective of the residents rather than focus on the personal lives of the staff members who raised the issue. This approach reinforced the idea that staff had a job to do and supported their dedication to do it well.

I reminded them that the primary issue for residents was safety. If staff members could establish their own responsibility for the safety of each resident, then the problem of cravings or resentment could be handled by specific interventions, such as the debriefing mentioned earlier. Residents would be informed at intake and reminded periodically that such an intervention would always follow a relapse episode. In this way, other residents did not have to fear that no one was really in charge, that the problem was going unnoticed, and that it would continue to happen. Then, depending on the particular culture and activities of each program, the staff might encourage a resident to share his or her story of relapse with other members of the community, again, with the goal of communicating a level of understanding about one's behavior, not as an opportunity to confront the individual. Confrontations would be handled as staff-mediated discussions at the request of any resident and would focus only on disruptive behaviors, not the offending person's drug use. This type of intervention, I believed, could help reduce residents' fears of other people's drug use.

Additionally, some residents complained, "You let someone else use. Why not me?" They felt that they were being held to a rule that others were allowed to break. In this situation, a twofold intervention could be designed. First, when residents entered the housing program, they were asked to make a list of the reasons why they stopped using drugs (or if still using, why they might want to stop). Then, whenever they voiced a complaint or a fear about using again, the staff could redirect them back to this document and help them answer their own question, "*Why am I* not using?"

## Recommendations Made to the Corporation for Supportive Housing

These consultations provided immediate assistance to agencies that needed to make some quick changes and started a process of programmatic development that would require nurturance and support. With this in mind, I made a few recommendations in two specific areas: staff development/training and program development.

Staff development/training could be provided by the funding agency's technical assistance personnel and/or outside consultants. This training would assist staff to resolve confusion and reluctance about the meaning of harm reduction as it applied to their program and to the entire system. In addition, staff from the Corporation for Supportive Housing could provide specific, small-group skills training in the areas of conflict negotiation, motivational interviewing, deescalation techniques, and community building.

In terms of program development, there is a clear need for a full range of housing opportunities, and efforts should be made to identify the particular strengths and culture of each program. While moving in the general direction of harm reduction will help to reduce the incidence of homeless in some groups of people, there will continue to be residents who use drugs and those who do not, those who are relatively tolerant and those who feel intensely threatened by drug activity near them. Since harm reduction is basically a philosophy of inclusion and choice, it is possible to offer a full choice of programs, some of which are more abstinence-oriented than others. The key is to communicate the culture of each particular program to prospective residents prior to their moving in by reviewing typical house policies regarding behavior. To have current residents meet with an applicant also helps to introduce the new resident to the expectations of the *community*, giving the applicant a better idea of how the program fits with his or her lifestyle. If there are other housing choices, applicants will most likely gravitate to a program that fits their needs. However, attempts to overly homogenize the system result in fewer quality services and more turnover of both staff and residents. Diversity of residents both within and between the programs helps to create communities where people can learn from and help one another.

## Conclusions

While this consultation project focused on the particular needs of staff and residents in housing services, the model can be used to effect change in other clinical and service settings as well. Once the staff assimilate the basic tenets of harm reduction, they are usually able to suggest concrete changes that best fit their agency. Outside consultation is useful to begin the process of change and may reduce staff feelings of powerlessness or helplessness in the face of significant client problems. Ultimately, however, it is the ongoing efforts of the program staff and clients that effect the most lasting change.

## GRAND ROUNDS CLINICAL
## CASE CONFERENCE

A different opportunity to apply the general model of harm reduction psychotherapy occurs in the area of clinical case consultation and clinical supervision. Since this model is multidisciplinary, it is particularly able to fit the needs of patients who present with multiple problems. The following section presents an example of how to use the model with a seriously disturbed patient who is enmeshed in a complex health system with multiple providers. The confusing nature of her symptoms, the high cost of treating such a patient, and the limited availability of intensive, individual treatment services could result in a potentially ineffective intervention strategy. The goal, therefore, is to create a treatment plan that is both effective and realistic in the current system.

This section begins with case information garnered from a patient within a community mental health setting. Following a review of background information, I discuss several important points relevant to diagnosis and treatment, including the need for tolerance of the patient's symptoms at the same time that symptom reduction remains a priority.

## Patient Information

This patient, Nina, a 32-year-old female of mixed African American and Native American background, identified strongly with her Hopi heritage and was somewhat disparaging of her African American roots. Since the age of 18, she had had a long history of involvement with social service and community mental health systems in the San Francisco Bay Area.

Nina was removed from her mother and father's care when she was a little over 1 year old, possibly for failure to thrive (a physical condition of poor growth related to both nutritional and emotional neglect). Both parents were alcoholic, and her father may also have been using marijuana. From ages 4–14, Nina was shunted through several foster homes until settling in at one. In this home, she was beaten by her foster mother and sexually abused by an older foster brother. She reported the abuse when she was 14 and was removed from that home and placed in a group home. Within a few weeks, she began to decompensate, expressing suicidal intent and cutting her arms and abdomen. While the details of her life at this time are vague, Nina says that she ran away to another city and managed to live on the streets by "scrounging." Within 6 months, however, she was picked up for public drunkenness and assault, and sent to a state hospital program, where she remained for 2 years. For the first 6 months during that hospitalization, she made numerous suicidal threats and engaged in self-injurious behaviors almost daily.

Released into the community as an emancipated minor, Nina moved in and out of shelters and psychiatric crisis units, unable to settle in stable housing or treatment. She had numerous intimate relationships with male drug dealers with whom she did drugs, including crack cocaine, alcohol, and marijuana. Over the past 4 years, Nina had had treatment in many programs: drug and psychiatric, residential and outpatient, dual-diagnosis, and traditional 12-Step groups. She had remained abstinent from crack cocaine for 3 years and used marijuana only occasionally, but she continued to drink large quantities of alcohol, typically in a binge fashion.

Of great concern were her near continuous suicidal impulses and self-injurious behaviors. Nina cut her arms and legs with knives and razor blades, producing large wounds that often required both stitches and tendon repair. She had one wound on her arm that she kept open by rubbing sharp objects into it. She became agitated and obsessively ruminated about harming herself. Only drinking or cutting herself had any ameliorative effect on her obsessive ruminations and affective flooding.

Despite such serious psychopathology, Nina's therapist saw several strengths in her patient. Nina had been able to work within a sheltered workshop environment and had expressed a wish to do so again. She was honest about her behaviors and her feelings, stating that alcohol was the only thing that took away her often overwhelming feelings of anxiety, dread, and rage. Even though her interpersonal relationships were chaotic, Nina no longer got involved with men who were violent with her, or who dealt drugs, and she maintained friendships with two or three women she met in shelters.

Several medical conditions complicated Nina's case. She had asthma, for which she used an inhaler. She was diagnosed with minimal brain dysfunction, but no details were available. Perhaps related to this, Nina complained of poor short- and long-term memory. She was obese (more than 20% over her ideal body weight), and suffered from primary hypertension. She had not menstruated in many years and had suffered numerous pelvic infections. She was HIV-negative.

The diagnostic impressions of this patient had remained stable over many years. Nina suffered from major depression, recurrent, severe; posttraumatic stress disorder; and borderline personality disorder.

At the time of this case consultation, Nina was in the hospital again and wanted to be released because she felt more agitated there than at her hotel.

## Case Discussion

The comments and treatment recommendations are intended both as case-specific and as general guidelines for this type of patient. I am aware that some of what might constitute optimal treatment is not available for patients like Nina, but alterations may be possible to approximate the most intensive interventions suggested.

- *I'm not convinced that her suicidality and self-injurious behaviors (SIBs) are depression-related.* While her symptoms are most characteristic of periodic borderline personality disorder decompensations, it could very well be that these symptoms are part of either a posttraumatic constellation that includes intense dysphoric affects or a psychotic depression, which would account for the obsessive, agitated quality to her presentation. Hints for differential diagnosis: How quickly does the dysphoric affect develop? Does she have any of the cognitive or vegetative signs of depression, either during these episodes or at other times? Are they related in any way to drug (stimulant) use or withdrawal? How quickly does the dysphoria abate as compared to the SIB ideation? It is important to assess the timing of the symptoms we are calling depression because, within this diagnostic category, in contrast to so many others, treatment does actually follow diagnosis. Because of their long latency for therapeutic effect, antidepressant medications do not typically work very well in reducing or eliminating storms of dysphoric affect that are acute and reactive in nature. Such a medication may, in some people, raise the threshold for the *expression* of this symptom, but the patient still experiences the painful emotions. If the person meets the criteria for major depression *in addition to* the SIBs and dysphoric affect storms, it may be worthwhile to begin a trial of antidepressants, keeping in mind that therapeutic response is often muted in borderline patients, who often experience more side effects than do others (Cowdry, 1987). A low dose of an antipsychotic medication is often very helpful to calm a patient who is experiencing an affect, or "borderline storm" (Gitlin, 1996; Soloff, 1987).
- *It makes little sense to require that she stop SIB and substance use as a condition for treatment or housing.* Nina has been terminated from treatment and housing situations before, and it has not "motivated" her to remain abstinent. Also, she clearly stated that she

felt alcohol was her tool for dealing with herself. Until this is addressed, she will remain motivated to continue drinking rather than to stop. Her current housing situation (residential hotel) is probably better for her than a residential treatment program, as staff there can tolerate the self-destructive behavior while clinicians work with her to curtail it. Requiring a person to stop this behavior usually results in treatment or placement failure.

• *This patient complains of feeling too "contained" in hospital; she feels she needs to get out and do something to numb out.* This is a typical pattern seen in SIB patients as opposed to borderline patients without significant self-injury patterns. It is also seen in juveniles with depression masked by acting-out behaviors. Nina may actually be getting more seriously suicidal while in the hospital. While what is being "contained" are the behaviors that worry *clinicians*, the threat that *she* feels is actually the content (the story) of the past abuse, current interpersonal stressors, and her attendant feelings. I would avoid dealing with the content while she is hospitalized. Contrary to some opinions, the hospital is generally not a safe place for her to deal with this material because her stay is too short term. On the other hand, I would name for her the process of how containment seems to increase her psychological tension and suicidality. The clinicians could offer her an empathic response regarding her use of alcohol to obliterate (contain) affect, while encouraging her to develop other means to decrease affective intensity.

• *Nina is probably right that the alcohol (and other drugs?) control or eliminate painful affects.* It is essential to honor the power of drugs to work for patients coping with negative affect states. Denying this, or stressing only the negative consequences, creates a situation where the patient has to agree overtly or resist, neither of which is good for the therapy. Nina is accomplishing several complex neurochemical changes with her various behaviors and drug use.

*Alcohol* causes the release of dopamine and GABA, which may create potent antidepressant and soothing effects. Alcohol is also causing disinhibition which allows Nina to act out the SIBs prior to experiencing the calming effects.

Her *cutting* can be seen as both a behavior and a drug. As a drug, it releases endogenous endorphins (those internal, opiate-like chemicals that create a feeling of soothing), even though the behavior itself recreates the original trauma and ultimately initiates her body's original defense against it.

*Stimulants* cause a rapid release of dopamine and norepinephrine, resulting in emotional soothing, mental alertness, and decreased depression. This assists Nina in her attempts to get away from painful affect states and temporarily relieves dysphoria. Stimulants do, however, increase impulsivity and quickly deplete norepinephrine, with a resulting severe rebound depression.

*Marijuana* may have antianxiety effects as well as produce a kind of cognitive "muddling" that may relieve intrusive thoughts and images. It may have paradoxical effects, however, and can eventually cause psychotic-like changes in cognition. With marijuana especially, patients are often not aware that the drug may be causing the very symptom they are trying to avoid.

The offerings from our pharmacies are generally no match for these potent drug effects, and the side effects of prescribed medications are often, subjectively, at least, worse for the patient.

• *Nina is also right that she cannot tolerate painful affects.* It is counterproductive for the relationship, as well as erroneous, to think that we can offer Nina some quick techniques for affect tolerance. The ability to tolerate affect is developmental and requires a combination of time, safety while expressing affect, teaching and limiting its expression, and the consistent presence of a soothing other. Chances are, this woman is not going to get much of this anytime soon. We can, however, teach her some affect avoidance or modulation techniques for the short run.

• *It is unclear to what degree a psychotic process underlies Nina's condition and to what degree it is a product of characterological decompensation.* The differential diagnosis of borderline pathology, schizotypal personality, and psychotic conditions continues to be difficult, despite the realization that borderline conditions do not in fact rest on any particular border. Treatment decisions often cannot be made based on an accurate diagnosis but may have to rest on a hierarchy of symptom clusters that more closely resemble one or another disorder. It is important to attempt to assess whether cognitive or affective symptoms predominate in this woman. Jerome Kroll (1988) addresses this problem as one of differential microdiagnosis and offers several treatment recommendations that follow from the assessment. In Nina's case, it appears that affective intensity and lability predominate, but her clear problems with affect may, in fact, be covering psychotic-like cognitive problems that appear when she is under stress (confusion, memory deficits, poor linear thinking).

## Treatment Suggestions: Harm Reduction in Action

With the preceding comments in mind, I formulated an outline of important considerations for designing a treatment program for Nina. This style of consultation is consistent with the general approach of harm reduction psychotherapy in that the individual methods of the primary therapist are respected and treatment is planned around the unique relationship between the patient and the therapist, and the attitudes, biases, and approaches that each brings to the psychotherapeutic relationship.

Nina presented with serious, life-threatening symptomatology that causes intense distress to clinicians and other providers. It is less certain that her overt symptoms cause *her* distress, even though she is obviously suffering emotionally. While her suicidality seems paramount, she actually has a moderate lethality index, based on prior behaviors, that shows no signs of increasing that I can detect. She may, of course, accidentally kill herself, either directly or as a result of infection, accidental injury, and so forth. It is always tempting to bring in the "big guns" of psychotherapy, such as involuntary hospitalization, forced medication compliance, and contracts against self-harm, when dealing with a patient who is so obviously a risk to herself.

I believe that it is usually a mistake to coerce such a patient into behavioral restrictions or treatment goals that have not been mutually established. Nina has spent the greater part of her life within the public health system and shows little interest in pursuing goals that we, as therapists, might see as necessary or beneficial. Whether willing or not, the community mental health system obviously has a long-term commitment to care for this type of patient. Palliative or punitive responses may result in increasing severity of symptoms and potential lethality. Providing only maintenance support services, such as case management and rehabilitative day treatment, is likely to result in increased suffering for the patient and her caregivers, and increased cost for the system. Nina needs ongoing individual psychotherapy in addition to sophisticated clinical case management services if her primary difficulties are to be resolved.

• *Nina gets relief from drugs and cutting herself. How can we mimic these effects while she is building emotional muscle?* Earlier in this section I briefly outlined some of the complex neurochemical events that Nina provokes by using drugs, alcohol, and self-cutting. Given that she needs immediate relief from her overwhelming affects, how could we help her gain similar chemical (and emotional) benefits using techniques that will cause less harm? Several strategies have been used in other clinical populations for the purpose of containment and relaxation, although very little research has been done on the efficacy of such interventions for patients with character pathology. The different practices include deep relaxation, distraction techniques, obsessive rituals that soothe or compete with other harmful rituals, and the use of prn (as needed) neuroleptics to the point of sedation in response to the patient's felt need to blur/wipe out intense feelings.

(The clinician must remember that while Nina is frightened by strong affect, it is still a part of her self that she identifies with and values. She may have an unconscious resistance to ridding herself of these strong feelings).

• *How exactly do I help a patient build emotional muscle?* First, identify a target feeling (patients like Nina are often alexithymic, so the therapist may need to provide a word such as "upset" or "angry"). Then, rate that particular feeling on scale of 1–10 (least to most intense ever experienced). Next, intervene, do something active, whether patient-initiated or clinician-mediated, to reduce the disturbing affect: medications, relaxation, distraction, conscious effort, suggestions offered when the patient is in a deeply relaxed state similar to a hypnotic state. Do not, however, hypnotize such patients. They are highly suggestible and fragile, and hypnosis often disinhibits strong feelings. In addition, hypnosis should never be used by someone who is not fully certified in its use. After the intervention, have the patient rerate her experience of affect intensity on scale of 1–10. Reinforce any tiny change and point out observed but not felt changes. Patients frequently fail to notice changes that others can detect. This is true for medication response as well as other behavioral and emotional changes. Repeat this process as needed with different feeling states.

• *Is there some way of putting Nina's drug use under medical control?* Since she is obviously using drugs at least in part to medicate on a prn (as needed) basis, could a psychiatrist help Nina titrate the alcohol and other drug use to her acute symptoms? This is a radical approach that may not be possible or even desirable in many treatment settings, but is nonetheless an important principle of harm reduction interventions. Right now, Nina is probably overusing alcohol in order to get a rapid effect of dissociation. She could probably get the same good effects from lower doses of alcohol but in the moment is too panicked to realize this. It might be helpful to get her to work with a physician and/or nurse to use prescription medications as well as alcohol or marijuana as prn (as needed) medication strategies that are directed by someone else (i.e., a medical professional), with input from her encouraged. Dosing schedules can be arranged for any psychoactive drug.

## Medication Strategies

Gitlin (1996) offers comprehensive advice on medication strategies for patients like Nina. It may be best to prescribe a low dose of an antipsychotic such as risperidone or Mellaril and teach Nina when and how to use it. It could also be beneficial to begin a trial of an SSRI at or above therapeutic doses to treat her obsessive symptoms and affective storms, and monitor for side effects that may affect compliance. The antidepressant Wellbutrin might be a good choice for some patients, since it is a dopamine-enhancing drug and Nina's use of alcohol and stimulants indicates that her brain may be craving dopamine. However, she may relapse on stimulants and therefore increase the risk of seizures with this particular medication. Wellbutrin could also cause an increase in psychotic-like thinking and, in any case, will not work for obsessiveness or rumination and may increase agitation. Despite the bad press, benzodiazepines such as Librium or clonopin work well for people like Nina. She should not use these as long as she is drinking, though. If she could ever be trusted with the antialcohol drug Anabuse, one could consider using such antianxiety medications as suggested earlier.

Finally, a discussion of the meaning of medications to a patient allows dynamic issues to be uncovered (Housner, 1993). Clinicians are often surprised to realize that many drug-using patients are very hesitant to take psychotropic medications. The clinician typically responds with some statement such as "Well, you're already using

drugs, and they aren't even of known quality." This response misses
the point. Many drug-using patients are very attached to their role as
the one providing relief for themselves. Allowing a doctor to be the
drug prescriber can raise concerns about being controlled or not being cared for sufficiently. In addition, the person knows how to get
relief quickly rather than having to wait for a clinical effect to take
place over time (with antidepressants, up to 5 weeks).

- *Find out why the patient quit the drugs that she no longer
uses.* This gives you insight into what kinds of things motivate her to
change. People are always motivated; they just may not be motivated
by what *we* want. Work with her to develop a decisional balance.

- *Remember, the mental health system is her family. She may
not want to grow up, that is, get better and "leave home."* Assess her
current status on the stages of change in terms of SIB as well as the
alcohol and other drug use. This allows the therapist to see what is
really motivating her either to get better or produce symptoms.

- *Ultimately what might work best for her is a group affiliation:
12-Step, church, or a cultural association.* With a continual source of
support, structure, and a feeling of family, but with complete freedom to come and go, Nina might find the best combination for herself. How did she relate to 12-Step models in other treatment programs? Ask specifically what she liked and did not like, what she
found helpful or not.

In terms of church, does she sing? How about the choir? Would
she like to help children or work on a special event at a community
center?

Nina identifies more as Native American (Hopi) than black. Native American associations offer many benefits to people like Nina.
Support and recognition of her ethnic identity can be a potent force
for change. The sense of community and of shared problems creates
the feeling of family that this patient will continue to need. In addition, these societies are more likely to understand the enormous variations in drug and alcohol use among different tribes (Westermeyer,
1996) and be better able to integrate her into their activities.

*       *       *

These two consultation projects are examples of the wide variety
of possible applications for harm reduction treatment models. Be-

cause such strategies derive their impetus from the immediate person, context, and culture, situation-specific interventions are more easily constructed and input from all people is valued. Just as the psychotherapy model is intended to be adopted into a clinician's existing orientation, so can consultation and training take advantage of existing staff and program strengths. It is my hope that many different versions of psychotherapy, program development, and public policy will develop from some of these ideas. It is through diversity of opinion and intervention that we can reach the largest number of people and reach out to them, with respect for their rights to live a healthy life.

## THE DIFFICULTIES OF COMBINING MODELS AND TECHNIQUES

Even though the techniques of harm reduction psychotherapy are varied and allow for the use of many different theoretical orientations, some will find it difficult to apply this model in their own practice. Many clinicians notice that, over time, their style of working becomes patterned. Whether a patient enters therapy for depression, anxiety, or relationship problems, many of us tend to use the same basic therapeutic stance and techniques. In this way, no matter what our theoretical orientation, many of us end up practicing a kind of eclecticism that is not necessarily well thought out. I am suggesting that in order to use the principles in this book, clinicians must develop a kind of "informed eclecticism" (Zucker, 1995), that is, a well-thought-out mixture of theories, approaches, and techniques that are flexible enough to work with a wide variety of patients, yet consistent enough to allow us to communicate our work to each other and give us a basis for self-evaluation. There are, of course, many different theoretical orientations. For the purpose of this book, however, I discuss primarily attitudes and techniques that are typical of some psychodynamic and humanistic practitioners, partly because this is the orientation with which I am most familiar, and partly because it is often an underlying orientation even when cognitive or behavioral techniques are used. Clinicians who are trained primarily in cognitive-behavioral models do not have the same difficulties. It is likely that these clinicians have more difficulty integrating work on the dynamics of attachment and less on technical considerations.

## Difficulties with Standard
## Psychotherapy Techniques

While psychotherapies in general tend to be respectful of the patient's perspective, there are a number of difficulties that arise from the fact that therapist training imbues clinicians with a certain "stance" that at times interferes with the kind of active helping required in work with drug users. This section speaks in generalities and, therefore, should not be construed to be a primer on all therapeutic models but, rather, a rough guide for clinicians to evaluate their practice as it applies to alcohol and drug abuse problems.

Many psychotherapies focus primarily on process rather than content. Indeed, surprisingly few therapists conduct a formal assessment inquiry, nor is a diagnosis necessarily established as a means to guide treatment. The day-to-day details of the patient's life are not routinely examined and may, in fact, be interpreted as resistance if the patient insists on talking about such details. It is just this kind of direct questioning and attention to details that is essential in working with drug use behaviors and problems (of course, the questions are asked within the guidelines of motivational interviewing).

Additionally, many therapies (not only psychodynamic, but also various "humanistic" forms of psychotherapy) focus on long-term "depth" or insight work rather than on present behaviors and symptoms. The assumption is that if the underlying emotional problems can be resolved, then the "symptom" of drug abuse will fall away. Such a stance is unnecessarily polarized: drug use may, in fact, be a symptom of underlying psychological problems, but once the drug use has become serious (dependence), the use develops a functional autonomy and becomes a "central activity" (Fingarette, 1988) that requires specific knowledge and interventions that are outside the usual expertise of psychotherapists.

This focus on process and insight results in a kind of therapy that leads to several typical stylistic as well as theoretical problems. Psychodynamic therapists tend not to develop overt goals and treatment strategies with patients. Many clinicians, then, when working with a drug abusing person, export this responsibility to other clinicians in order to preserve the supposed neutrality of the primary therapeutic relationship. The resulting split does not, in fact, preserve therapeutic neutrality; rather, it forces patients to straddle different expectations and different relationships in a way that often mimics their childhood experiences. In a more integrated approach, the primary therapist would be centrally involved in the articulation of goals and strategies, even if certain interventions were within the purview of other providers.

This concern about a split treatment model is extremely confusing. While the primary therapist needs to be more active, it is often important to use several other treatment providers as well. One area of confusion is the issue of group therapy and self-help groups. Most psychotherapists are not trained in group psychotherapy and do not know how to assess a patient's readiness for it. Some clinicians are developing specific guideline for incorporating harm reduction into group psychotherapy (Little, in press). Many therapists, though, are often unaware of the exact nature of groups, whether therapeutic or self-help with the result that many clinicians are afraid of possible splitting and prefer to keep the relationship safe from outside interference. In my experience, a good group therapist is a lifeline for me as well as an additional support for my patient. The more people involved in the care of someone with severe addiction problems, the better the potential for lasting change. Open communication is important, of course. But we need to recognize that what we term "splitting" is often merely patients' attempts to attend to all aspects of their personality. We do not all have to agree in order for treatment to be effective. Open communication of differences allows patients to retain the important role as the final arbiter of their treatment and their lives.

The area of neutrality has come under scrutiny within the psychodynamic field. In terms of addiction work, the use of therapeutic neutrality tends to underestimate the impact of cultural biases on the self-esteem of the patient. A noncommittal stance by the therapist is all too easily interpreted (rightly or wrongly) by the patient as a negative judgment. Of course, such projections are at the heart of psychodynamic treatment, but in areas of cultural or political sensitivity, such projections are not necessarily the workings of a distorted psyche, but the assumptions formed by lifelong experience. In addition, since the clarification of values is at the heart of the decisional balance, ignoring such moral concerns, or offering no guidance in the patient's quest for what is right or wrong, is of very little help.

There is yet another consideration regarding therapeutic neutrality. If a therapist finds drug use and drug users abhorrent, it might be better to refer these patients rather than adopt an attitude of neutrality, as these types of values tend to be communicated to the patient in many subtle ways by the therapist. Walant (1995) cautions that neutrality may hide yet another countertransference reaction, that is, the therapist's discomfort for, or disdain of, the addict's need to experience moments of merger, of intense closeness, during the therapy. Many therapists have been trained to see the need for "immersive" moments as regressive and to value only separation/individuation. This stance prevents the active emotional movement toward the patient that contributes to healing.

A related area that may cause some therapists discomfort is the level of activity that is required during parts of the treatment using harm reduction psychotherapy. We have been trained not to give advice out of a desire to avoid gratifying our patients' dependency needs, and we make few distinctions regarding how legitimate those needs may be in a given person's treatment. Skills training requires a kind of personal involvement and advice giving that some may worry is intrusive or infantalizing. Other clinicians, who believe that insight is what causes behavioral change, prefer not to offer specific suggestions that might be useful in the moment. Still others are hesitant to raise a new topic in the therapy, preferring instead to wait for "an opening." Such passivity is not possible during certain phases of addiction treatment. The patient needs to focus on certain thoughts, feelings, and behaviors, and the therapist needs certain information. Oftentimes, this cannot wait for the patient to "get around to it."

Working with the transference can sometimes become a competitive issue in this treatment. While we tend to use the transference between patient and therapist as the focus for many interpretations and much reparation, it is often the transference relationship between the patient and the drug that is of primary importance, especially early in the treatment. We have to keep in mind that the person is preoccupied with this primary attachment figure (alcohol or drugs) and may have little psychic energy for a relationship with a therapist. Some therapists inaccurately label this phenomenon as "resistance to the transference." It is humbling to realize that we are not, after all, the most important object to our patients.

Finally, with some patients, it is important to be actively involved outside of the usual therapeutic frame. Phone contact is one example. Most clinicians reserve phone contact between sessions for emergencies only. With some patients, however, it is very useful to offer phone contact at particularly difficult times of the day or week. I have set aside time around the end of the workday to talk with people who are having trouble avoiding "cocktail hour." Others call in the morning, when they are used to taking speed to get themselves going each day, sometimes just to leave a voice-mail check-in. This type of availability can make the difference between a successful therapy and one full of setbacks.

## THE COST OF TREATMENT AND THE NEED FOR SELF-HELP SUPPORT GROUPS

The previous recommendations for extra contact highlight a significant difficulty in applying this model within large-scale practices or agencies. Because most medical insurance will not cover outpatient therapy for drug or alcohol problems, or because those that do often require that the patient be enrolled in an "official" treatment program, the cost of the treatment is usually borne by patients and their families. In addition, the time that it takes to respond to phone requests for contact, or merely to listen to messages, is prohibitive if one has a full practice. At this time, there are not enough self-help groups available except for 12-Step meetings. Some of my patients do take advantage of these meetings, but most of the patients that I see came to me specifically because they wanted a treatment that did not use 12-Step methods. I can sometimes facilitate the use of both approaches by a patient, but it does not work very well unless the person has some openness to 12-Step methods. Going to meetings for support but not choosing a sponsor or working the steps is a compromise for some patients. There are some professionally led groups that offer nontraditional treatment, but many more are needed in order to provide a peer support system for patients who need it.

Perhaps those who "mature out" (Peele, 1991) of substance abuse problems can shed some light on this dilemma. Clearly, those people who have resolved their alcohol or drug problems without the help of 12-Step or treatment programs have employed some strategies that worked for them. They did, in effect, create a individualized self-help program that may have included family members, social networks, religious affiliations, and civic organizations. We, as professionals, need to expand our definition of self-help beyond drug- or alcohol-specific groups to include these other important sources of support for our patients. The essential goal is to create an inclusive community, one in which people with drug problems can be exposed to the competing values and personal connections that could help them resolve their addictions. This expansion of support opportunities and the inclusion of drug users within regular societal institutions will decrease the demonization of drug users, increase the strength of the community, offer 24-hour support to those who need it, and, ultimately, create a path out of drug or alcohol addiction.

Despite these difficulties, more harm reduction approaches to psychotherapy can be developed that focus on the needs of different types of patients in a range of treatment settings. The movement toward truly client-centered treatment embraces all orientations. It is my hope that the reader can find useful ideas and tools from this book and begin, or continue, to develop treatments within his and her own community.

## ETHICAL CONSIDERATIONS AND INFORMED CONSENT

It is a serious enterprise to develop a new treatment model, especially one that diverges from the existing professional paradigm as much as this one does. These ideas are likely to be received with more than the usual amount of interest, ambivalence, or dismissal, as are new ideas in other areas of psychology. After all, drug treatment in this country involves social and political issues, and legal statutes, in addition to psychological theory and research. Nonetheless, I have attempted to take into consideration all the factors that are involved in the design of new treatment models. I want my treatment model to conform to the principles of ethics established the American Psychological Association (1992). These ethical guidelines require extensive training in areas that are new to one's practice and recognize that in newly emerging professional areas, one might not be able to get formalized training. In order to ensure that I was following this ethical code, I undertook both formal (a Diplomate-Fellow certificate in psychopharmacology) and informal (reading and consultations) training tasks. I wrote this book partly to give such a training tool to other clinicians in order to create a professional community that specializes in harm reduction approaches. Many of the authors cited in this book have contributed greatly to the development of this area and to my own development as well. I recommend that readers make use of the extensive bibliography to begin their own training.

The recent findings of Project MATCH (1997) lend support to my belief that many different treatments are effective for alcohol problems. While not a study of harm reduction methods per se, I did find some interesting results in this area. Project MATCH examined three different types of alcohol treatment, 12-Step facilitation, cognitive-behavioral coping skills, and motivational enhancement therapy. Results showed that all were equally effective as primary treatments, although none of them was hugely successful (only about one in four persons maintained sobriety throughout the year-long study). The most robust outcome was the reduction in total amount of alcohol drunk and in several areas of alcohol-related harm. While abstinence was the internal goal of the treatment, researchers were heartened to find that the treatments did some good even for those who did not remain abstinent, concluding that different treatments are successful in harm reduction goals.

Since harm reduction appears to be the most likely outcome of abstinence-based treatments, the practice of using harm reduction goals at the inception of treatment aligns actual practice with research results. One does not know, however, which patient might do better with an abstinence goal and which will not. Will allowing patients to select moderation as a treatment goal merely postpone the eventual necessity of abstinence? And what if significant harm accrues to them or to society in the meantime? There are no easy answers to these questions, and this lack of clarity determines one's clinical comfort level. Allowing clients to dictate their own goals about how they want to live their lives may create incapacitating anxiety in the therapist. If this is the case, the therapist should not attempt to do this kind of alcohol and drug treatment. Rotgers (1998, pp. 69–70) offers an excellent discussion of this countertransference dilemma.

Another ethical consideration is the requirement for informed consent for treatment. This process actually clarifies for both patient and therapist the exact nature of the treatment decisions that are be-

ing made, and by whom. Clinicians are bound to offer treatments accepted by their professional peers as the "standard of practice."
However, *all* of the treatment options should be discussed, including
the relative risks and benefits involved in each of the choices. Options for moderation should be discussed, including the relative pros
and cons from the therapist's point of view:

> "I understand that you would like to continue using heroin, but
> not every day. Since you have only been using small amounts
> and have only been using for a few months, that may be a possi-
> bility for you. On the other hand, you have already been ar-
> rested once and may not want to take that risk again."

Of course there is another possible scenario:

> "You think you would like to continue drinking, but just not so
> much at one time. You could certainly try to do this, and there
> are some techniques that may help you; however, you have been
> drinking heavily for 20 years, and you have a high tolerance
> level. The research that we have suggests that, for someone with
> your drinking history, trying to cut down is not likely to be suc-
> cessful in the long run. You might be able to reduce your drink-
> ing to safer amounts, but it's likely not to last for more than a
> few months or so."

This informed consent discussion clearly lays out the possibilities
and what is or is not known from research or clinical consensus. It
must be clear to both the patient and to the clinician that the ultimate
choice is made by the *patient*. The therapist recommends *neither* abstinence or moderation but gives information and helps patients clarify what they want to do. I generally put this discussion in writing,
adding also that some newly developed harm reduction methods are
not considered the "standard of practice" in the field. Five years
from now, I hope to be able to add more specific information to the
consent discussion, but until then, I will be guided by a combination
of collegial input, research, and experience.

*APPENDICES*

# APPENDIX A

---

# Overview of
# Psychoactive Drugs

$\mathbf{D}$rug actions are governed by the principles of *pharmaco-kinetics* and *pharmacodynamics*. Psychoactive drug actions (drugs that act within the brain and result in mood changes) are caused by the drug's direct influence on neurotransmitters and/or other actions in the brain. All of the following information refers only to drugs that are psychoactive, not general medical drugs such as those taken for infections, regulation of blood pressure, and so forth. A bibliography follows the description of drugs, so that the reader may continue to learn about how drugs work.

Pharmacokinetics refers to how the body acts on the drug—the journey of the drug through the body. There are four basic processes: absorption, distribution, metabolism (biotransformation), and excretion.

*Absorption* refers to the route of administration (how one takes the drug) and includes routes such as oral ingestion, nasal inhalation, smoking, and intravenous injection. These different routes are important in that they cause different degrees and rates of absorption. For example, oral ingestion (e.g., a pill) requires that the drug pass through the stomach acids, then into the intestines for absorption. It then goes to the liver, where some or all of it may be destroyed before it even gets to the brain. Intravenous injection, on the other hand, enters circulation directly and

205

generally bypasses the liver, avoiding the *first pass effect* that destroys so much of the drug. Smoking a drug allows it to enter arterial circulation immediately, thus affecting the brain almost instantaneously. The route of administration affects the addiction potential of a drug. In general, the faster the route, the higher the addiction potential.

*Distribution* refers to the movement of the drug past cell membranes, into organs and tissues. All psychoactive drugs are distributed to the brain; thus, they must be lipid (fat) soluble to cross the blood–brain barrier. (Lithium is an exception. It is not fat soluble and does not enter the brain.)

*Metabolism* refers to the processes in the liver that break down drugs into their component parts via enzyme activity. These parts, called metabolites, are then rendered water soluble for the next process, which is *excretion*. Most psychoactive drugs are excreted by the kidneys in the form of urine.

Pharmacodynamics refers to what the drug does to the body, how it exerts its effect. This is usually referred to as the *mechanism of action* (MOA). *This abbreviation should not be confused with another, MAOI, which stands for monoamine oxidase inhibitor, a type of antidepressant medication.* All psychoactive drugs share a similar MOA in that they affect central nervous system activity either directly or through the effects of neurotransmitters on synapses. The primary neurotransmitters are dopamine (DA), norepinephrine (NE), serotonin (5-HT), gama-aminobutyric acid (GABA), and glutamate. It may be that all drugs produce euphoria secondary to dopamine release in several areas of the brain (mesolimbic dopamine pathways such as the amygdala, hippocampus, anterior cingulate, nucleus accumbens, and the ventral tegmental area).

Drugs cause both short- and long-term effects in the brain. In general, short or irregular use of a substance causes direct action on the neurotransmitters, either increasing or decreasing their activity. Regular or prolonged use, however, also causes structural changes to take place as a result of alterations in the genetic material, messenger RNA, of the nerve cell. These changes may result in tolerance (when one must take more of the drug to get the same effect) and physiological dependence.

An important term in pharmacodynamics is *half-life*, which is shown by the symbol $T_{1/2}$. This refers to the length of time it takes for the body to metabolize half of the dose taken. In general, the shorter the $T_{1/2}$, the higher the addiction potential (e.g., in the brain nicotine has a $T_{1/2}$ of about 25 minutes, cocaine about 20 minutes, some amphetamines about 4 hours).

The addiction potential of any drug is related to both the route of administration and the half-life. The faster the route and the shorter the half-life, the higher is the addiction potential (smoking cocaine vs. taking a narcotic pill).

All drugs are presented in the following format:

1. Popular name(s)
2. Chemical/generic name
3. Pharmacodynamics (MOA and effects)
4. Pharmacokinetics
5. Physiological consequences (short and longer term)


## ALCOHOL

**Popular Names:** Booze, juice, hooch.

**Chemical/Generic Name:** Ethyl alcohol or ethanol (ETOH).

**Pharmacodynamics:** ETOH depresses synaptic transmission in the brain by facilitating the GABA system, which is an inhibitory system responsible, in part, for relaxation. The cerebral cortex is the first part of the brain that is affected, which results in disinhibition (subjective feelings of relaxation, mild euphoria). With higher doses, the next to be affected is the cerebellum, causing slurred speech and an unsteady gait. With much larger doses, the medulla may be affected, causing respiratory depression and eventual death. In some people, euphoria is replaced by "the blues" or anger. Excess use causes vomiting in most people.

**Pharmacokinetics:** ETOH is absorbed in both the stomach and intestines. (The first ounce is absorbed via an active transport mechanism in the stomach.) The drug is distributed throughout the body, including passing the blood–brain and placental barriers. By-products of the metabolism of alcohol are toxic. The liver transforms ETOH first into acetaldehyde (which is toxic) by the enzyme ADH (alcohol dehydrogenase), then into acetate, which is inactive and goes into the Krebs cycle, where it is burned for energy. The rate of metabolism is about one ounce of pure ETOH per hour (see Chapter 3 for approximate amounts). Heavy, prolonged drinking leads to the use *of alternate metabolic pathways:*

> *Microsomal ethanol oxidizing system (MEOS)*—this type of enzyme induction leads to tolerance, because ETOH is more rapidly metabolized even though ADH itself is not induced.

*Catalase*—cofactor with hydrogen peroxide.

## Physiological Consequences of Long-Term Use:

*Psychiatric*—sleep disorders, anxiety, depression.

*Nutritional*—poor diet is not the only cause; vomiting, diarrhea, malabsorption, and interference with nutrient metabolism may occur; B-complex vitamins and minerals most affected; Vitamin C only somewhat affected.

*Cancers*—oral cavity and larynx, especially if also a smoker; liver, possibly colon.

*Trauma*—death by violence and accidents (60% of drivers in fatal crashes; 54% of fatal burns; 40% of all emergency room patients; 86% of homicides, rapes, family violence; 48% of suicides).

*Specific Organ Systems*:

*Nervous system*—Korsakoff's syndrome, a late occurring, chronic dementia and Wernicke's syndrome, which is acute and caused by a thiamine deficiency.

*Other nervous system*—peripheral neuropathies, dementia, necrosis, cognitive deficits from functional interference with protein synthesis, sleep disorders.

*Liver*—hepatic encephalopathy (ammonia), sudden onset mental status changes; Stage 1: fatty liver—uses hydrogen for fuel instead of fat (common); Stage 2: alcoholic hepatitis—cell destruction occurs (not common); Stage 3: alcoholic cirrhosis—cells die and are replaced by fiber, which causes chemical changes and mechanical blockage.

*Digestive system*—irritant to mucous membranes, gastritis, pancreatitis, malabsorption syndromes.

*Blood*—anemia, leukopenia.

*Heart*—cardiomyopathy (muscle becomes fat and fibrous and enlarges; leads to congestive heart failure. Hyperlipidemia leads to arteriosclerosis).

*Fetal alcohol syndrome*—severe retardation, characteristic structural features.

*Withdrawal Syndrome:* Generally starts 6–8 hours after last drink. Diabetic coma and organ rejection mimics it.

*Stage 1*—tremulousness, restlessness, appetite loss, insomnia, anxiety, apprehension, elevated pulse and respiration. This is the most common type of withdrawal.

*Stage 2*—tremors become more severe, shaky feeling inside, anxiety and dread increase, along with pulse and respiration. Alcoholic hallucinosis may occur.

*Stage 3*—Delirium tremens (DTs). Serious and life threatening. Terror, hallucinations that are tactile as well as visual and auditory, alarming increase in blood pressure, fever, grave mental status changes (orientation), possible seizures.

*Medical detoxification:* The goal is to prevent DTs and seizures. A history of prior withdrawals is important. There are generally four steps to managing withdrawal:

1. Good nursing care (titrate medications to hand tremor).
2. Mild antianxiety or antihypertensive agents—Vistaril, Inderal.
3. Single dose of Valium or Librium.
4. If needed, escalate dose of Librium (50 mg Librium now, then 25–50 mg every 30 minutes as needed (prn) for tremulousness with a maximum dose of 300 mg. The goal is to produce mild sedation. Decrease the dose on the second day and discontinue by the third day.

## DEPRESSANTS (OPIOIDS)

**Popular Names:** Smack, junk, horse, dillies, Number 4's

**Chemical/Generic Names:** Heroin, codeine, opium, morphine, meperidine (Demerol), propoxyphene (Darvon).

**Pharmacodynamics:** Analgesia, sedation, cough suppression, antidiarreal, smooth muscle relaxant, euphoric. Those that are rapid onset/ short duration most often abused (heroin and Demerol). Morphine and heroin are poorly absorbed by mouth. Opioids depress neuron firing especially in pain pathways. Opium alkaloids are agonists; they interact with endogenous beta-endorphin and enkephalin receptors in pain pathways, the substantia gelatinous, the limbic system, and the hypothalamus.

**Pharmacokinetics:** Rapidly absorbed by intramuscualar or intravenous injection. Poorly bound to plasma protein, does not accumulate in tissues, metabolized by liver, excreted through bile and the kidneys.

**Physiological Consequences:** Mostly from poor hygiene, poor quality control (presence of adulterants), dirty needles, general lifestyle. Hepatitis B and C, tuberculosis, tetanus, cellulitis and abscesses, HIV, "cotton fever," Mexican brown dementia. The opioid drug itself causes little or no long-term damage to the body, except for constipation, which can be dangerous if severe.

*Overdoses*: Occur primarily when tolerance has decreased after a period of abstinence or in a novel situation. The person then takes the old usual dose, which can cause respiratory and cardiac arrest.

*Tolerance*: Accommodation on a cellular level; high accommodation to euphoria, analgesia, nausea, respiratory depression; mid accommodation to slowed heartbeat; little accommodation to pupil constriction, constipation.

*Dependence*: Cells accommodate to a disruption of homeostasis. Drug replaces naturally occurring brain peptides.

*Withdrawal Syndrome*: Similar to a severe case of the flu. Within 8–10 hours after last dose, the person will experience yawning, sweating, runny nose. After 48–72 hours, peak of symptoms; insomnia, violent yawning, sweating and goose bumps (cold turkey), muscle and joint pain. After 7–10 days, symptoms stop, but may get a protracted withdrawal of another 1–3 weeks in which the person shows marked intolerance of stress, discomfort, changes in temperature. Severe low self-image as well.

## DEPRESSANTS (NONOPIOIDS)

**Popular Names**: Barbiturates—blue devils, yellow jackets, reds; nonbarbiturates—goofballs, ludes, soapers.

**Chemical/Generic Names**: Amobarbital (intermediate acting), pentobarbital (short acting), methaqualone.

**Pharmacodynamics**: Similar effects as ETOH. These are central nervous system depressants that cause a euphoric feeling leading to sedation, with a very small window in terms of blood levels. These drugs also have antiseizure and muscle relaxation properties. Decrease sleep latency for up to 14 days.

**Pharmacokinetics**: The drug is absorbed by the small intestine and has a rapid distribution and onset of action. Metabolized by liver; 100% absorbed, 40% protein bound.

**Physiological Consequences**: Depression, irritability, weight loss, possible nutritional problems. Dependence and tolerance develop rapidly and they are cross-tolerant with ETOH. Rapid deterioration of cerebral and liver functions can result from extreme use over a short period of time.

*Withdrawal Syndrome*: Extremely dangerous. Rebound effect lowers seizure threshold with possible status epilepticus. Insomnia results from REM sleep rebound and leads to irritation and anxiety.

## STIMULANTS

**Popular Names**: Cigarettes, coffee, chocolate, crack, coke, snow, bennies, crank.

**Chemical/Generic Names**: Nicotine, caffeine, cocaine, amphetamines, meth-amphetamine, methylphenidate (Ritalin).

**Pharmacodynamics**: Central nervous system stimulation via blocking the reuptake of serotonin and norepinephrine; ultimate depletion of these neurotransmitters. Positive effects include euphoria, confidence, elation, increased mental alertness and focus, appetite suppression, increased motor and speech activity. Some of the negative effects are restlessness, irritability, weight loss, psychosis, and spasms of neck, mouth, and jaw muscles.

**Pharmacokinetics**: Rapidly absorbed by intestines, lungs, intravenously, all mucous membranes. If oral route, is first partially metabolized by liver; if not oral route, drug bypasses this "first pass" effect and goes directly to the bloodstream. Can be found in pancreas, spleen, kidneys. Stimulants, like other psychoactive drugs, are metabolized by the liver.

**Physiological Consequences**: Nasal tissue damage, posthigh depression, amphetamine psychosis, possible irreversible brain damage, seizures, cardiac arrest, stroke, severe nutritional deficiency, hypertension.

*Dependence*: Highest danger with shorter acting drugs (crack).

*Tolerance*: May not develop in all people or with all varieties of stimulants.

*Withdrawal Syndrome*: Extreme depression with acute suicidality possible, fatigue, drug craving.

## ANXIOLYTICS

**Popular Names**: Valleys, blues.

**Generic/Chemical Name**: Benzodiazepines.

**Pharmacodynamics:** Enhances the action of GABA (inhibitory neuro-transmitter) by binding to specific receptor sites. Relief of anxiety, muscle tension, mild euphoria, and relaxation are sought-after effects.

**Pharmacokinetics:** Metabolized by liver. Different varieties range from short- to long-term half-life, depending on plasma binding and active metabolites (Halcion vs. Valium); 100% absorbed and distributed throughout the body and brain.

**Physiological Consequences:** The shorter acting drugs tend to cause the most problems for people. These drugs can cause confusion in the elderly and decrease motor skills in all ages. Long-term use may interfere with learning new material.

*Dependence:* In general, the use of two to three times a therapeutic dose for 6 months will result in physical dependence. The shorter acting drugs, however (such as Halcion) may cause dependence in as short a time as 1 month in some people.

*Tolerance:* One tends to develop rapid tolerance to the sedative effects of these drugs, necessitating increasing doses if being used as a sleep agent. However, one does not tend to develop tolerance to the antianxiety effects when used regularly.

*Withdrawal Syndrome:* May be mild or severe, with possible seizures 4–10 days after last dose (10 hours after last Halcion). Insomnia, irritability may last for as long as a month. Latent phase possible after 3–4 months. General rule is to do a very long, very slow taper off the drug, first substituting a longer acting one for a short acting one.

## CANNABINOIDS

**Popular Names:** Grass, weed, hash, bhang, hooch, ganja, joint, reefer, dope, pot, dooby.

**Chemical/Generic Names:** Marijuana, hashish, Kif, charas, THC, Bhang (beverage).

**Pharmacodynamics:** Relaxation, euphoria and the "giggles," slight tremors, increased sensitivity, increased appetite and heart rate, alteration in sense of time, impairment of judgment and coordination. Dry mouth and eyes. (Some people feel paradoxical effects of nausea, dizziness, acute anxiety.) Properties of both stimulants and depressants, but is neither, nor is it a true hallucinogenic. Prolonged use diminishes the alterations but not the relaxation.

*Medical Usage*: Control of nausea and vomiting, asthma (in small doses), glaucoma, muscle relaxation in cases of brain injuries and multiple sclerosis. Many people say it reduces menstrual cramps, headache. The less frequently one smokes marijuana, the more medical benefits the patient is likely to get.

**Pharmacokinetics**: Disputed. The main chemical, THC, resembles no other known psychoactive molecule. It is insoluble in water, but very soluble in oil. Stays in the body a long time and is stored in body fat.

**Physiological Consequences**: With long-term use: lethargy, anhedonia, lack of motivation (amotivational syndrome), possible psychotic-like changes in cognition, sterility in males, possible immune dysfunction, respiratory irritation (pot has more tar than cigarettes).

*Addiction*: Tolerance does develop with daily, heavy usage. Cutting back, even for a few days, will reduce tolerance. Dependence can occur with newer, high-dosage pot. Physical symptoms of withdrawal are not medically significant but can be psychologically significant and distressing. Adaptation can be significant, meaning that a user can learn to perform motor skills well and not have depressed reflexes.


## HIGHLIGHTERS/SCRAMBLERS (PSYCHEDELICS
## AND AMPHETAMINE PSYCHEDELICS)

**Popular Names**: Acid, donna, the racer's edge, angel dust, MDA, MDMA (Ecstasy or Adam).

**Chemical/Generic Names**: LSD, peyote, belladonna, STP, multiple amphetamines, MDMA, PCP.

**Pharmacodynamics**: Scramblers cause intense visual and perceptual changes or hallucinations. Sensory switches and heightened sensitivity are prominent. Autonomic/sympathetic nervous system: Some people experience intense fear or paranoid reactions. Behavioral dyscontrol is possible. MDMA ( Ecstasy or Adam) is noted for its very specific effects and lack of true hallucinations at usual dosage. It seems to enhance certain mental functions: emotional ecstasy, empathy, serenity, self awareness. Reports of dopamine or serotonin reduction have not been proven.

**Pharmacokinetics**: Absorbed through the small intestine. Half-life ranges from short (30 minutes for DMT) to long (12 hours for LSD, and 24 hours for DOM). Metabolism is assumed to be via the liver, but little is really known.

**Physiological Consequences:** Possible psychotic-like changes. Memory disturbances. Acute terror reactions. Possible metabolic and neurological changes with PCP. These drugs are not thought to cause physiological dependence but can cause intense psychological dependence.

## INHALANTS AND DELIRIANTS (SOLVENTS, ANESTHETICS, VASODILATORS)

**Popular Names:** Poppers, pearls, locker room, rush.

**Chemical/Generic Names:** Amyl nitrate, butyl nitrate, other deliriants (nightshade, mushrooms, nutmeg). Some authors include PCP and ketamine.

**Pharmacodynamics:** Inhalants such as amyl nitrate dilate arteries, resulting in a sudden fall in blood pressure, a throbbing feeling in the head, warmth and flushing of the skin, and dramatically altered state of consciousness. Deliriants cause profound mental status changes and are highly unstable in terms of their effects. PCP, a dissociative anesthetic, is an unstable compound that can cause unpredictable and uncontrollable rage, paranoid reactions, and superhuman strength. Scopolamine is the active chemical in many of these drugs. Ketamine (vitamin K), is also a dissociative anesthetic, but its effects are more predictable, including increased energy, lack of awareness of physical pain, disinhibition. May be potentially fatal when combined with alcohol.

*Physical Effects:* Include parched mouth and burning thirst; hot, dry skin; feverish feeling; inability to focus at close range; rapid heart rate; constipation; ejaculation difficulties in men. Half-life is different for each drug, ranging from 30 minutes to several hours.

*Mental Effects:* Include restlessness, vivid and horrifying hallucinations with amnesia for the experience, disorientation that can cause serious injury. Long history of use by criminals and herbalists, and in Native American male initiation rituals.

**Pharmacokinetics:** These drugs are rapidly absorbed by inhaling, smoking, injecting, ingesting. Transported quickly to the brain and some may stay in body tissues. Metabolized by the liver, often with serious medical consequences.

**Physiological Consequences:** Delirium, dementia, damage to the cerebellum (affecting gait and proprioception). Acute paranoia and violence (especially with PCP). Major trauma resulting from accidents caused by a total dissociation from reality.

## APPENDIX B

# References for Specific Drug Effects

American Psychiatric Association. (1995). Practice guideline for the treatment of patients with substance use disorders: Alcohol, cocaine, opioids. *American Journal of Psychiatry, 152*(11; Suppl.).

Bezchlibnyk-Butler, K., & Jeffries, J. J. (1998). *Clinical handbook of psychotropic drugs* (8th ed.). Seattle: Hogrefe & Huber.

Inaba, D., Cohen, W., & Holstein, M. (1997). *Uppers, downers, all arounders* (3rd ed.). Ashland, OR: CNS Publications.

Kuhn, C., Swartzwelder, S., & Wilson, W. (1998). *Buzzed: The straight facts about the most used and abused drugs from alcohol to ecstasy.* New York: Norton.

Medical Economics Co. (1998). *Physicians' desk reference* (52nd ed.). Montvale, NJ: Author.

Nestler, E. (1995). Molecular basis of addictive states. *Neuroscientist, 1*(4), 212–219.

Schuckit, M. (1989). *Drug and alcohol abuse: A guide to diagnosis and treatment* (3rd ed.). New York: Plenum.

Snyder, S. (1996). *Drugs and the brain.* New York: Scientific American Library.

Stahl, S. M. (1996). *Essential psychopharmacology: Neuroscientific basis and practical applications.* New York: Cambridge University Press.

Stimmel, B. (1997). *Pain and its relief without addiction: Clinical issues in the use of opioids and other analgesics.* New York: Haworth.

# History of Drugs and Attitudes toward Them

*I*t is all too common in the field of mental health to minimize the influence of history and culture on the way people behave, how it affects the way we categorize behaviors as normal or deviant, and how we respond to them. This gap is especially prevalent in the area of drug use. Our attitudes toward alcohol and other drugs do not, of course, have a purely individual or professional origin. It is naive to assume that political, social, and religious forces have no power over our most closely held beliefs and no influence on our theories. As therapists, we must be careful that our work stays separate from our private life, where bias and prejudice are our prerogative. Without offering a comprehensive history, the next section traces the general trends, attitudes, and laws regarding alcohol and drugs in the United States. The changes in our attitudes over the past 200 years provide an insight into U.S. culture as it developed.

Alcohol, usually in the form of beer and other malt beverages, was used by people of all cultures, from ancient civilizations to modern times. In medieval and renaissance England, the daily allotment of beer was 1 gallon per day for every man, woman, and child (Manchester, 1992). The reasons for this practice most likely included the euphoric effects of alcohol, its pain killing properties, and the uncertain water quality that was found in ponds and slow-moving streams. Drugs, of course, have an equally long history of use, particularly in religious ceremonies and in the shamanic tradition.

There have been several paradigm shifts in how we view persons who abuse alcohol or drugs. Even though drugs and alcohol are companion issues, it is helpful to separate them, because the use and meaning of drugs and alcohol have taken separate courses in U.S. history. Alcohol in particular has had a contradictory course. We have not always assumed that regular, even heavy, drinking constitutes a problem. Europeans who settled America brought with them their habits of drinking (Conroy, 1991). Other drugs were introduced in America primarily as medicinal tonics and herbal preparations—touted as cures for just about every ailment—that were heavily laced with narcotics and alcohol as well.

With the exception of certain religious sects, Colonial Americans drank heavily. Occasional bad behavior was tolerated, but habitual drunkenness was seen as a sign of moral weakness. This belief marks the beginning of the controversy about the causes of addiction. During different points in the history of the United States, the alcoholic has been seen by some as evil, by others as morally weak, and, since the 1950s, as having a biological disease. All of these attitudes placed people addicted to drugs or alcohol in a category separate from others, unable to be understood by the general principles of human behavior prevalent at the time. Currently, the premise of addiction as a disease informs the field and the popular view. How did this happen?

## ALCOHOL IN THE UNITED STATES

It is interesting to note that there has always been a debate about alcohol in the United States. Fundamentalist Christians deplored drinking, but as North America was colonized by more diverse groups, the national consensus appeared to be that alcohol was a regular, normal part of the culture. As socioeconomic and political conditions changed, however, so did the apparent consensus. Temperance organizations brought the debate about alcohol use back to the public eye, and many people became convinced that alcohol was indeed an evil spirit. This led to the prohibition of beverage alcohol for 13 years. Since then, the national consensus has returned to the belief that alcohol consumption, when moderate, is a normal part of life for many.

Colonial Americans brought with them the culture of England and Western Europe. Conroy (1991) describes these times in great detail. Barrows and Room (1991) add many fascinating facts as well. Central to this culture was the local community tavern that operated not only as an establishment for food and drink but also as a center of community life. Town meetings were held in the taverns, business was conducted, and families lingered there during the long cold winter evenings as a way of conserving fuel. Any occasional lapse into drunken behavior was duly noted and commented on by one's neighbors, and this peer pressure was generally enough to keep bad behavior in check. This acceptance of alcohol in everyday life changed over the course of years and resulted in two groups with opposing attitudes toward beverage alcohol.

In general, fundamentalist Protestants deplored all drinking. These people, originally in the Northeast, eventually inhabited rural America, the South, and the Midwest. Other Christians, Jews, immigrants, city dwellers, and various liberal coalitions saw alcohol as an important part of their culture and enjoyment of life. These disparate views coexisted until around 1826, when groups of Protestant women began the Public Hygiene movement, aimed at improving the health of foreign immigrant workers and protecting the rest of the population from diseases that were epidemic in the urban ghettos. These women ultimately formed the basis of the temperance and anti-saloon movements that resulted in the ratification of the Eighteenth Amendment to the Unites States constitution. Prohibition began in 1920 (Tyrell, 1991). The Women's Christian Temperance Union was the most visible crusader organization, followed by Carry Nation and the Anti-Saloon League.

The concept of temperance quickly turned into a public policy of abstinence for all. Why? From 1785 through the mid-1800s, a large segment of U.S. society changed from a tightly knit, local community tavern lifestyle, to industrial, isolated, urban living. Immigrant families were particularly displaced, isolated, and missed the supportive extended family structure of the "old country." The cultural boundaries and injunctions for proper behavior no longer existed, and people's lives were disrupted. At about the same time, the westward expansion filled the prairies with single men, unmoored from the general bounds of society, who were creating a new culture, that of the cowboy, a rough-and-tumble loner who came into town to drink and fight.

This era also saw the end of community regulation of problems and the beginning of government interventions (e.g., asylums, poorhouses). Public drunkenness became an extreme problem in urban working-class society and in frontier life. Women and children were beaten by drunken husbands; mothers left their children to fend for themselves while they got drunk after returning from the factories. It was in this climate during the Industrial Revolution that the temperance movement began to see alcohol as dangerous to everyone, an uncontrollable habit that must never be started. (It is noteworthy that this is the current public attitude toward narcotic use). Women were visibly active in the temperance movement because they, as wives and mothers, suffered the most from widespread alcohol abuse. Their best interests would be served if their husbands were bringing home their wages instead of spending them at the tavern. By 1855, over one-third of the states had prohibited alcohol.

Many other people were involved in the discussion about alcohol. As early as 1785, Benjamin Rush developed the idea that the key element of this dangerous affliction of drunkenness was a disease that caused loss of control over how much one drinks (Fingarette, 1988). The Moral Re-Armament movement of the 1930s offered a solution—religious conversion. The Washingtonians, and later the members of the all-male Oxford group, were major temperance organizers. Conversion, admission of powerlessness over temptation, public confession of wrongdoings, and public service were the key steps toward recovery from sinfulness, and salvation. It was assumed that spiritual growth, including abstinence from alcohol, was the key to social and political change. In addition to their stance on alcohol, many of these groups were antiforeigner, anti-Catholic, and antiliberal. One of their political slogans was that Democrats were the party of "Rum, Romanism, and Rebellion!" (Bufe, 1991; Fox, 1993).

This worry about rebellion (unionizing) not only affected the factory owners of the industrial North but also was a major concern of slave owners in the South. The role that alcohol played in slavery was complex and disturbing. Alcohol was often given to male slaves as part of a "freedom" celebration after long stretches of work. The slave owners hoped to pair the idea of freedom with the feelings of hangovers and thus reduce the chance that their slaves would rebel or run away. On the other hand, some slave owners punished drinking with public lashes. These contradictory approaches were quite effective, and formed the basis for the post–Civil War involvement of African Americans in the abstinence movement. However, subsequent exposure to racism within the movement caused black people to withdraw their support long before Prohibition came into effect (Herd, 1991).

The most extreme voices rose in the United States when Carry Nation formed the Anti-Saloon League in 1895. This group engaged in tactical preventive actions such as torching and demolishing saloons throughout the country with a vehemence reminiscent of today's religious and political terrorists. The activity of these groups resulted in the enactment of a Constitutional amendment prohibiting the sale of alcohol. Prohibition had the unfortunate effect of giving rise to organized crime and, paradoxically, resulted in heavy drinking for many people. The speakeasy became a social scene for the sole purpose of drinking, unlike the saloon era, when people gathered for other purposes. Lack of quality control caused serious medical problems. Most illegally available alcohol came in the form of distilled spirits rather than the lower potency beer and wine previously consumed in the United States. The result was greater levels of intoxication and more serious medical problems associated with drinking. Methanol, or wood alcohol, was legal and cheaper than ethanol (beverage alcohol), and was routinely mixed with beverage alcohol. Too high concentrations of methanol resulted in many medical problems, including blindness (hence the term "blind drunk").

Prohibition ended in 1933 but the attitudes of people toward alcohol could not change overnight. If alcohol was so dangerous that it had been banned, how to explain the lifting of that ban? It was in this climate that the disease model was developed and Alcoholics Anonymous (AA) was started (Bufe, 1991; Fingarette, 1988). Two men, Bill Wilson, and Bob Smith (Dr. Bob), members of a social–political association called the Oxford Group, suffered from alcoholism and wanted to help other people like themselves. They took the standard Oxford philosophy and spiritual program of the Moral Re-Armament movement (admission of sinfulness, public confession of wrongdoing, conversion to a Christian life that includes public service to others not yet saved), and developed a self-help model wherein freedom from addiction is accomplished by rigorously following 12 specific steps. They created meetings for alcoholics in hopes that what had helped them in their battle with alcoholism would help others. They wrote *Alcoholics Anonymous* (fondly called *The Big Book*) in 1939 as a guide to the AA program and life without alcohol. Bill and Dr. Bob (as they are referred to in the program) asserted that alcoholism affects only a special group of people who are unable to control their drinking because of some biological factor. Alcoholism is inbred and therefore irreversible.

American ambivalence about alcohol is still a live issue. Europeans look at us with incredulity, as their attitudes toward drinking have changed very little, so there is almost no public debate. Ethnic, religious, and regional groups differ greatly in abstinence rates; in general, the countries with the highest rates of abstinence also have the highest rates of alcoholism (note that countries with high rates of drinking, while having generally lower rates of alcoholism, do tend to have a higher incidence of alcohol-related medical problems). The percentage of abstainers in the United States (over 45%), equal to that in Ireland, is the highest in the Western World. The United States has a 15% incidence of alcoholism in a culture where 45% of adults are abstinent. Ireland, Scotland, and Denmark have similar or higher rates, whereas France, Italy, and Israel have lower rates of alcoholism and few adult abstainers.

## OTHER DRUGS

Narcotics were introduced as medicines in the late 1700s, long before there was any concept of addiction to explain the phenomenon of people needing to take higher doses over time and becoming sick when they stopped using the tonic. The typical user at this time was a white, middle-class woman taking tonics for a variety of "female" problems, including weakness, fainting and headaches, and menstrual pain. After taking these tonics for a while, a woman would become ill if she stopped. It was assumed that this illness was a return of the previous symptoms for which the tonic was first given; thus, the obvious medical intervention was to resume taking the tonic. The concept of physical dependence or addiction was not applied to these cases.

During the Civil War was the first time that massive addiction occurred and spilled over into the general public. Soldiers were given morphine for battle wounds and returned home with the "soldier's disease," which was, of course, what we now think of as the withdrawal syndrome. This sparked the search for a nonaddictive painkiller that continues to this day. Chemists, pharmacists, and physicians were eager to discover an effective and safe alternative to morphine. The irony of this effort is that it resulted in the manufacture of several narcotics that were even more addicting than morphine! Heroin, synthesized by the Bayer company in the 1890s and touted as the cure for morphine addiction, was a central ingredient in cough remedies. Demerol, a synthetic narcotic, was soon followed by the development of methadone in 1950.

Opium, the original plant narcotic from which others were synthesized, was seen as an essential part of a physician's treatment for many disorders and later was used by intellectuals in the United States and Europe. The nonnarcotic plant marijuana was considered the poor man's opium. Cocaine was thought to be medicinal *and* a tonic. It was included in most herbal remedies as well as in Coca-Cola. Many professionals, most notably Sigmund Freud and his colleagues, used cocaine in large quantities and gave it to their patients as well (Walant, 1995). After a time, it became clear that cocaine was severely addicting and caused a toxic psychosis characterized by tactile hallucinations, called the "cocaine bug."

Over time, it has become apparent that culture plays an important role in the use of mind-altering substances. Excessive use often occurs when a drug or substance is first introduced, as if the culture has not yet had time to develop social norms for its use, or is mistaken about its effects. Abuse problems often result. Coffee was thought to be a dangerous foreign drug in Europe in the 1600s. Secret societies were formed to drink the strong beverage in coffeehouses after dark to avoid arrest. The result was widespread addiction and toxic psychosis from the caffeine, a high-potency stimulant drug (Weil & Rosen, 1993).

In Jewish culture, wine has been available since ancient times. It is used both socially and for ceremonies and rituals, but Jews in general have a very low rate of alcoholism.

It is important to note that in the United States, attitudes toward drugs have often been intertwined with the complicated legacy of racism. In the 1850s, Chinese laborers arrived in San Francisco and brought with them their habit of smoking opium. Economic and political agendas were often couched in racial prejudices to influence the population to change the laws regarding use of these drugs. Posters depicting Chinese men in San Francisco, high on opium, and black men in the South, high on cocaine, assaulting white women, fueled a hysteria that resulted in national legislation that banned the *smoking* of opium in 1909 and cocaine in 1914.

The laws regarding drug possession and use have a long history in the United States. It is beyond the scope of this book to give the details regarding the sequence of legal changes and the sociopolitical climates within which they occurred. Musto (1987) offers a comprehensive discussion of this topic.

The typical narcotics user, who was a white, middle-class female, remained constant until the Harrison Narcotics Act of 1914 banned opium and cocaine. Tonics were outlawed. With this legislation, drug use moved from white, middle-class, middle-aged women to poor people supplied with illegal drugs by criminal elements. Middle- and upper-class women had originally used narcotic tonics heavily laced with alcohol and cocaine, then barbiturates, and finally benzodiazepines such as Valium. But after the passage of another legislation, the Comprehensive Drug Abuse Prevention and Control Act of 1970, which set up a schedule of drugs based on supposed medicinal value and abuse potential, the profile of the drug user and addict changed significantly again. Physicians grew more reluctant to write prescriptions for controlled substances, partly because of their own changing attitudes, and partly as a result of intense surveillance and reporting efforts by government agencies. Once aware of the dangers of barbiturates and benzodiazepines, the medical community also began to limit the amount of these drugs prescribed at any one time. Women and middle-class people reduced their use of these drugs as well. However, they still use the majority of *legally prescribed* drugs. Racial and economic minority groups did not significantly reduce their use, however, and have since formed the core of the illegal drug users in this country. Without a private physician to prescribe drugs, these users turned to dealers instead. Today, middle-class people tend to take prescription painkillers or diet pills and drink alcohol. Poor people of color take heroin and cocaine, and have fewer problems with alcohol (Substance Abuse and Mental Health Services Administration, 1996).

During the years between the passage of these two laws (1914 and 1970), racial minorities were the primary users of illegal drugs, until the 1960s, when mostly young, middle-class people started using again. Stiffer penalties went into effect in the 1970s, and the use among middle-class whites, although still higher than minority use, declined again. The idea that the legal climate affects the demographics of illegal drug use is open to much speculation. It is possible that middle-class people are less compelled to use drugs and more controlled by the dominant legal culture than are poor people of color. It is more likely that drug use is driven by social and economic factors as well as the psychologically devastating effect of racism. It is interesting that while the rate of alcoholism is lower among blacks than whites, the rate of addiction to illicit drugs is reversed in these two racial groups. The social, economic, and racial factors in drug use are the source of much debate in the United States today.

# Self-Help Reading List

Bufe, C. (1991). *Alcoholics Anonymous: Cult or cure?* San Francisco: See Sharp Press.

Dorsman, J. (1991). *How to quit drinking without AA.* Newark, DE: New Dawn.

Ellis, A., & Velten, E. (1992). *When AA doesn't work for you: Rational steps to quitting alcohol.* Fort Lee, NJ: Barricade Books.

Forrest, G. G. (1989). *Guidelines for responsible drinking.* Northvale, NJ: Aronson.

Horvath, A. T. (1998). *Sex, drugs, gambling, and chocolate: A workbook for overcoming addictions.* San Luis Obispo, CA. Impact.

Kern, M. F. (1994). *Take control now! A do it yourself blueprint for positive lifestyle success.* Los Angeles: Life Skills Management.

Kishline, A. (1994). *Moderate drinking: The moderation management guide for people who want to reduce their drinking.* New York: Crown.

Knaus, W. (1998). *SMART recovery: A sensible primer* (3rd ed.). Longmeadow, MA: Author.

Levin, J. (1991). *Recovery from alcoholism: Beyond your wildest dreams.* Northvale, NJ: Aronson.

Miller, W. R., & Munoz, S. A. (1982). *How to control your drinking: A practical guide to responsible drinking.* Albuquerque: University of New Mexico Press.

Norcross, J. C., Santrock, J. W., Campbell, L. F., Smith, T. P., Sommer, R., Zuckerman, E. (2000) *Authoritative guide to self-help resources in mental health*. New York: Guilford Press.

Peele, S. (1991). *The truth about addiction and recovery*. New York: Simon & Schuster.

Pluymen, B. (1996). *The thinking person's guide to sobriety*. Austin, TX: Bright Books.

Prochaska, J., Norcross, J., & DiClemente, C. (1994). *Changing for good*. New York. Avon Books.

Sanchez-Craig, M. (1993). *Saying when: How to quit drinking or cut down*. Toronto: Addiction Research Foundation.

Trimpey, J. (1992). *The small book* (rev.). New York: Dell.

Washton, A., & Boundy, D. (1989). *Willpower's not enough*. New York: Harper Perennial.

Weil, A., & Rosen, W. (1993). *From chocolate to morphine*. Boston: Houghton Mifflin. (Original work published 1983)

# *Alternative Self-Help and Professional Resources*

SMART (Self Management and Recovery Training)
24000 Mercantile Road, Suite 11
Beachwood, OH 44122
National: 216-292-0220
Fax: 216-831-3776
*SRMail1@aol.com*
*http://www.smartrecovery.org*

SOS (Secular Organizations for Sobriety, or Save Our Selves)
SHARE Building, 5521 Grosvenor
Marina del Rey, CA 90066
National: 310-821-8430
*sos@directnet.com or sos@unhooked.com*
*http://www.unhooked.org*

WFS (Women for Sobriety, Inc.)
PO Box 618
Quakertown, PA 18951-0618
National: 215-536-8026 or 800-333-1600
*WFSobriety@aol.com*
*http://www.mediapulse.com/wfs*

RR (Rational Recovery)
Rational Recovery Systems, Inc.
Box 800
Lotus, CA 95651
National: 530-621-2667 or 530-621-4374
Fax: 530-622-4297
*rr@rational.org*
*http://rational.org/recovery*

MM (Moderation Management)
Moderation Management Network, Inc.
PO Box 1752
Woodinville, WA 98072
Phone: 425-483-5293
*mm@moderation.org*
*www.moderation.org*

MM online group discussion:
MM listserv. Send the following e-mail message with no subject line
to:
*listserv@maelstrom.stjohns.edu*
SUBSCRIBE MM YOUR NAME

On-line list of therapists who do MM:
*http://cybertowers.com/selfhelp/articles/atd/atdmoderate.html/*

Behavioral Self-Control Program for Windows (BSCP-Win)
Review: *http://www.ex.ac.uk/~mhnbrisco/cimh/bscpw.html/*
Order from: Reid Hester, PhD
3810 Osuna Road NE, Suite 1
Albuquerque, NM 87109
National: 505-345-6100
*www.lobo.net/~rhester/software.htm*

Addiction Treatment Alternatives
423 Gough Street, Suite C
San Francisco, CA 94102
Phone and fax: 510-893-5520
Phone and fax: 415-252-0669
*atapatt@earthlink.net*

(Dr. Patt Denning developed this psychotherapy model for addictions.
Individual and group psychotherapy, consultations, and training for
professionals in harm reduction and psychotherapy. Offices also in
Oakland.)

Addiction Alternatives
A division of Life Management Skills, Inc.
Beverly Hills Medical Tower
1125 South Beverly Drive
Los Angeles, CA 90035
310-275-5433
*habitdoc@msn.com*
*http://www.addictionalternatives.com*

(Dr. Marc Kern is the director of Addiction Alternatives. This private treatment agency offers a wide variety of self-help and professionally directed treatment options, including behavioral self-control training, computer-assisted recovery, mood management, and referral resources for legal and medical information.)

Practical Recovery Services
Dr. A. Thomas Horvath
8950 Villa la Jolla Drive
La Jolla, CA 92037-1705
858-453-4777
858-453-5222 Tape-recorded information about drop-in groups:
*info@practicalrecovery.com*

(Dr. Horvath offers a full range of outpatient treatment options, using cognitive-behavioral, rational, and other modalities.)

# Specific Treatment Modalities/Techniques

This appendix describes the basic principles of several different treatment types. It is possible to mix elements of several models, which is the approach in the cases in Chapter 5. Each brief description includes an important reference so that the reader can study the approach more carefully.

## COGNITIVE-BEHAVIORAL

Cognitive and behavioral perspectives on addiction have supplied the only other commonly known (and used) therapeutic models in this country. A number of specific theories and strategies exist in the literature. Additionally, most relapse prevention programs make extensive use of this type of conceptualization. It is difficult, indeed, to conduct drug treatment without using at least some of the techniques that come from this perspective. Three examples are behavioral self-control training (Hester & Miller, 1989), solution-focused treatment (Berg & Miller, 1992), and relapse prevention (Marlatt & Gordon, 1985). The first two programs were designed specifically for people with alcohol problems, but relapse prevention can be used with drugs, alcohol, or any behavior.

Hester and Miller's (1989) behavioral self-control training (BSCT), which can be used with abstinence or moderation goals, may be therapist-directed or client-directed by using a self-help manual. The program consists of implementing specific practices in an orderly way. First, clients set limits on the number of drinks they will have per day and per week to keep blood alcohol concentrations (BACs) at reasonably safe levels. This is done after clients have been educated about the effects of alcohol at certain BACs and over time. While Hester and Miller acknowledge that there are no clear guidelines for what constitutes a safe level of alcohol consumption, they note that exceeding three drinks per day is associated with increased health risks (Saunders & Aasland, 1987). Next, clients are taught to self-monitor their drinking behaviors and to begin to slow down the rate of drinking, as well as learning drink-refusal skills. As the treatment progresses, clients are taught to reward themselves for achieving their drinking goals, for recognizing triggers to drinking, and for developing other coping skills. This treatment has been extensively evaluated for effectiveness. Some guidelines are possible to implement. For those people who choose a moderation goal, an inability to significantly reduce their drinking within 6–8 weeks of treatment generally indicates that they will be unable to do so with more treatment and that abstinence is the best choice. This treatment works best for women and those drinkers whose problem drinking is of shorter duration and who have less physiological dependence.

Another program uses a strategic model in which client and therapist jointly construct a view of the client's problem and the possible solutions. This solution-focused treatment (Berg & Miller, 1992) is based on the following principles and assumptions: The emphasis is on mental health, highlighting the person's strengths and resources. In this framework, one looks for what is *right* with the client and how to use it (not what is wrong and how to fix it). The treatment tends to make use of current skills rather than teaching new ones. Berg and Miller insist that change is inevitable. One must identify naturally occurring changes and use them as building blocks. Most clients think that a problem is a constant. The therapist must help identify which behaviors are *not* a problem so that the clients can focus on their strengths.

Berg and Miller adopt an atheoretical/nonnormative client determined view that makes no assumptions about the *true* problems associated with abuse, only what is true for the individual. Finally, they rely on the law of parsimony, which dictates that one starts with the simplest assumptions regarding the nature of the problem and adds complexity to the treatment only as needed. This type of treatment utilizes a present and future orientation rather than a focus on past problems.

This treatment approach is resolutely practical and optimistic. It also requires, however, that the person be cognitively intact and have good verbal abilities. In addition, clients with serious psychopathology, or those whose lives are otherwise chaotic, may have difficulty following through on suggestions offered during the hour.

An important contribution of this approach is the designation of three types of client–therapist relationships. The *customer* type is represented by the client whose complaint or goal of treatment can be easily identified jointly by client and therapist. The client sees him- or herself as part of the problem. The *complainant* type, however, sees no connection between himself and possible solutions, and does not see himself as part of the problem. He may describe a complaint or a goal, but not identify any steps to take that solve the problem. Finally, the *visitor* type cannot identify a complaint or goal. Often these people are sent by others for treatment. They may complain of vague problems that are unrelated to the referring problem of alcohol abuse. Understanding these types is useful for a therapist in deciding on an approach to take with a client. If the client is not obviously a customer, Berg and Miller suggest finding the *hidden customer* in the difficult client by realizing that she may be willing to work on some other issue, such as decreasing pressure from someone else or stabilizing her housing situation. Keep in mind that the real customer may be the referring person. This approach is consistent with building a needs hierarchy, as suggested earlier.

Marlatt and Gordon's (1985) classic work, *Relapse Prevention*, has formed the basis of many different treatment modalities and approaches. This approach is derived from social cognitive theory, which is a combination of cognitive and social psychology, with a behavioral component. This broad theoretical and research base makes relapse prevention applicable to many different types of problems, and it can easily be used by a wide range of clinicians. It rests on several key assumptions: Addictions have multiple causes and consist of learned maladaptive coping responses to life's stressors and problems. Marlatt and Gordon also assert that addictive behaviors exist on a continuum rather than as an all-or-nothing phenomenon. Their research findings point not only to the importance of specific skills and clinical techniques but also to the essential role of developing a healthy, balanced lifestyle that is resistant to stress (resiliency).

The model consists of helping the individual identify and cope with high-risk situations, including the covert antecedents that often lead to risky situations. The clinician then helps the person alter some of the determinants of relapse, which include low self-efficacy, easy availability of drugs, and the perceived positive gratification of using. One of the most interesting and useful concepts is termed *AVE*, the abstinence violation effect. This is an emotional and cognitive response to violating a rule one has set for oneself, whether it be abstinence or moderation. The AVE response consists of self-blame and a feeling of being out of control, both of which cause self-efficacy to decrease, thereby increasing the chance that a lapse (a single instance of violating a rule) will become a full-blown relapse.

The relapse prevention model has often been construed as being useful only after abstinence has been established. It is just as useful, however, for working with clients to identify triggers, even if clients are still using, because the experiences are often fresher in memory and clearer than months afterwards. In ATA, just as in the assessment process, relapse prevention is intimately interwoven into treatment.

## PSYCHODYNAMIC PSYCHOTHERAPIES

All psychodynamic theories of addiction stress people's vulnerability to addiction because of preexisting emotional problems that prevent successful adaptation to adult life. These theories focus on the importance of affect, impulses, trauma, and conflict in the development and maintenance of addictions and usually apply equally well to both alcohol and other drugs.

Wurmser (1978) describes the prototypical addiction pathology as a narcissistic crisis that stems from the harshness of the person's superego rather than from a superego deficit. Using a drug temporarily overthrows the superego, quiets the internal critical voices, and allows a temporary liberation from guilt and rage. However, the diluting of the superego's condemning aspects is accompanied by a reduction in other functions as well, most notably self-esteem and self-care. Wurmser cautions therapists to avoid taking the role of the punitive parent, colluding with the patient's harsh superego. Rather, therapists should be supportive and neutral regarding the patient's drug use while exploring its meaning.

Khantzian (in Levin & Weiss, 1994) discusses addiction from the viewpoint of self psychology, a deficit model that differs from Wurmser's conflict model. He believes that addiction is an attempt to fill up psychological holes such as poor self-concept, poor self-regulatory functions (including affect regulation), and poor self-care. He also pays attention to the pharmacology of the particular drug of choice, stating that persons gravitate to a certain drug because of the particular feelings that they are trying to gain or manage. Khantzian, with this *self-medication hypothesis,* is the only psychodynamic clinician to address the actual drug of choice in any systematic way. Yet he, too, asserts that difficulties in affect regulation and tolerance are common to all addicts. His treatment consists of modified dynamic group therapy (MDGT), which emphasizes the underlying characterological issues that are universal among addicts.

Krystal and Raskin (in Levin & Weiss, 1994) offer another unique perspective on the difficulties of affect tolerance in addicts. They note that these patients have a characteristic "alexithymic" condition, lacking the ability to decipher the meanings of affects, experiencing them instead as physical states for which they have few descriptive words. This leads to poor coping strategies and the urge for discharge rather than understanding. Krystal and Raskin (1970) also see disturbed object relations and the resulting pathological structure of the self as being responsible for the characteristic impairments of addicts: poor self-care and self-control. To them, addiction is a variant of borderline personality organization, with its affective and impulsive problems. Krystal recommends that specific attention be paid to affect activation, that is, the development of both expression and labeling of feelings. He describes therapeutic techniques to develop modulation and tolerance of affect as well.

McDougall (in Morgenstern & Leeds, 1993) sees addiction as a psychosomatic problem in which persons disperse distressing feelings rather than identifying and thinking about them. The symbolic representation of feelings is a developmental phenomenon that somehow buffers strong emotions. Because addicts have not developed this ability to give inner elaboration to affect states, they are vulnerable to being overwhelmed by feeling states, and so discharge these "in action," as infants do. McDougall (1982) details the similarities between patients with clear psychosomatic problems and those with addictions, and makes extensive use of countertransference phenomena as a guide to her patients' internal states during treatment.

## SELF-HELP MODELS

These interventions are not actually treatment modalities in that they arise from an individual's need to find nonprofessional perspectives and/ or more extensive support than is available from formal treatment programs or clinicians. Many of these self-help models offer written materials, workbooks, and so forth. Others also include face-to-face group meetings and extensive social support. Most of these approaches can be integrated into psychotherapy, but the therapist should be aware of the general principles and biases of the different groups in order to deal with the patient's resulting conflicts or confusion of loyalties.

## 12-Step Groups

The best known self-help group is Alcoholic Anonymous (AA) and its more recent offshoots such as Narcotics Anonymous (NA) and Cocaine Anonymous (CA). These groups use a 12-Step process that is based on spiritual development as well as abstinence from substances. Twelve-Step groups are meant to be self-help groups that support persons both in their goal of abstinence and their spiritual development. Members typically attend groups, read literature, and meet with an individual sponsor to help them understand and "work the program" (follow the 12 Steps). In the United States, over the past 15 years, the philosophy of these groups has become the dominant paradigm for therapeutic orientations and treatment programs. As I have noted elsewhere, it is rare to find any chemical dependency treatment program that does not rely primarily on the tenets of the 12-Step model. These groups offer practical advice to cope with cravings and a community of people who have a firsthand understanding of the nature of addiction (withdrawal, recovery, and relapse).

On the other hand, psychotherapists sometimes criticize 12-Step approaches because the program is applied universally, with no acknowledgment of the importance of individual differences in the addictive process. This may cause difficulties in a psychotherapy in which the unique dynamics of the individual are the focus of discussion.

## Life Skills Enhancement

A good example of a self-help life skills approach is Stanton Peele's Life Skills Program (Peele, 1991). Peele has been a vocal opponent of traditional disease model approaches to the understanding and treatment of addictive disorders (Peele, 1991). His most recent book presents an alternative self-help model. His work can be used by individuals in a self-help framework or in individual or group therapy modalities. The general principles of the Life Skills Program include a belief that effective therapies are basically pragmatic rather than theoretical (or ideological), focused on concrete results rather than on the adoption of a new identity as an addict, and holistic in terms of considering the entire life of the patient and not just the addictive behaviors. Peele is adamant about the necessity of strengthening basic inter- and intrapersonal skills in the real world rather than segregating the person in groups of addicts. The workbook consists of a series of screening devices to help people assess the areas of strengths and weaknesses in their general life (friendships, job, hobbies, and interests). While Peele asserts that addictive behaviors can be controlled via the development of values and life skills, he takes no position on whether abstinence is required; thus, his approach can be used for a variety of patients. He does, however, criticize the disease model concepts of loss of control, denial, and inevitable progression. For patients who are not necessarily opposed to 12-Step methods but would rather use some other self-help approach, it might be wise to use ideas from his book (Peele, 1991), rather than the entire book, since the first part of the book is a scathing critique of traditional disease model treatments.

### Rational Recovery and SMART

There are a few other self-help group programs available in the United States. Rational Recovery (RR), originally based on the rational-emotive therapy of Albert Ellis, has undergone significant changes in the past few years. Developed by Jack Trimpey, it was originally conducted as a peer self-help group with professional advisors and now has changed to a professionally led method that also relies heavily on a workbook. The tenets remain essentially unchanged, however. The treatment is based on a belief that addicts have the power to control their behavior but often fail to do so because of deeply entrenched, irrational beliefs. *The Small Book* (Trimpey, 1992), a reference to AA's *Big Book*, is a guide for participants. A major difference between RR and 12-Step groups is that in RR, there is no set "program" to follow. Members are expected to figure out their own way to change their drug-use behavior. Another significant difference is that RR expects people to make limited use of the support groups, eventually leaving to continue their recovery in the real world and not needing continued work on the topic. Recovery is thus seen as a limited, accomplishable goal unlike the lifelong recovery of 12-Step programs.

The more recent *SMART* program, based on similar principles, is also professionally led.

### Secular Organizations for Sobriety (SOS), Moderation Management, and Women for Sobriety

These and other similar self-help groups are beginning to emerge across the United States as true alternatives to 12-Step meetings. All offer peer support; some, like Moderation Management, have professional leaders as well; some are informal, others are structured. A few of them are not abstinence-based. They offer all of the advantages of peer support without the necessity of following a spiritual program or accepting a role of powerlessness over addiction. The main difficulty is that there are so few of these groups meeting that they do not yet have the capacity for daily support in most cases. Therapists could offer support to these groups by giving patients information and resources to start their own chapters locally.

These are just a few of the many treatment approaches that use adaptive theories. Each therapist can find a model that fits with his or her own theoretical orientation or build new versions of traditional approaches. The use of consultation and a group of peers for discussion and support is a great help when attempting to develop a new treatment approach.

# References

Adelman, S. A., & Bar-Hamburger, R. (1994). The developmental grid technique for teaching the self-medication hypothesis of addiction. *Substance Abuse, 15*(1), 39–46.

Ainsworth, M. D., Blehar, M. C., Waters, E., & Wall, S. (1978). *Patterns of attachment: Assessed in the Strange Situation and at home.* Hillsdale, NJ: Erlbaum.

Alcoholics Anonymous. (1976). *Alcoholics Anonymous* (3rd ed.). New York: AA World Services. (Original work published 1939)

Alexander, B. K. (1987). The disease and adaptive models of addiction: A framework evaluation. *Journal of Drug Issues, 17*(1), 47–66.

American Academy of Addiction Psychiatry. (1996). *American Journal on Addictions: Special Series: Returning to Our Roots, 5*(2), 97–143.

American Psychiatric Association. (1987). *Diagnostic and statistical manual of mental disorders* (3rd ed.). Washington, DC: Author.

American Psychiatric Association. (1994). *Diagnostic and statistical manual of mental disorders* (4th ed.). Washington, DC: Author.

American Psychiatric Association. (1995). Practice guideline for the treatment of patients with substance use disorders: Alcohol, cocaine, opioids. *American Journal of Psychiatry, 152* (11, Suppl.).

American Psychological Association. (1992, December). Ethical standards of psychologists. *American Psychologist.*

Anthony, J. C., Warner, L. A., & Kessler, R. C. (1997). Comparative epidemiology of dependence on tobacco, alcohol, controlled substances, and inhalants: Basic findings from the national comorbidity survey. In G. A. Marlatt & G. R. VandenBos (Eds.), *Addictive behaviors: Readings on etiology, prevention, and treatment* (pp. 3–39). Washington, DC: American Psychological Association. (Original work published 1994)

Barrows, S., & Room, R. (Eds.). (1991). *Drinking: Behavior and belief in modern history.* Berkeley: University of California Press.

Berg, I. K., & Miller, S. (1992). *Working with the problem drinker: A solution-focused approach.* New York: Norton.

Bezchlibnyk-Butler, K., & Jeffries, J. J. (1998). *Clinical handbook of psychotropic drugs* (8th ed.). Seattle: Hogrefe & Huber.

Bower, B. (1997). Alcoholics synonymous: Heavy drinkers of all stripes may get comparable help from a variety of therapies. *Science News, 151,* 62–63.

Bowlby, J. (1982). *Attachment and loss: Vol. 1. Attachment* (2nd ed.). New York: Basic Books.

Bowlby, J. (1988). *A secure base: Parent–child attachment and healthy human development.* New York: Basic Books.

Brunswick, A., Messeri, P., & Titus, S. (1992). Predictive factors in adult substance abuse: A prospective study of African American adolescents. In M. Glantz & R. Pickens (Eds.), *Vulnerability to drug abuse* (pp. 419–472). Washington, DC: American Psychological Association.

Bufe, C. (1991). *Alcoholics Anonymous: Cult or cure?* San Francisco: See Sharp Press.

Chen, K., & Kandel, D. (1995). The natural history of drug use from adolescence to the mid-thirties in a general population sample. *American Journal of Public Health, 85,* 41–47.

Chiauzzi, E., & Liljegren, S. (1993). Taboo topics in addiction treatment: An empirical review of clinical folklore. *Journal of Substance Abuse Treatment, 10,* 303–316.

Conroy, D. (1991). Puritans in taverns: Law and popular culture in colonial Massachusetts. In S. Barrows & R. Room (Eds.), *Drinking: Behavior and belief in modern history.* Berkeley: University of California Press.

Cowdry, R. W. (1987). Psychopharmacology of borderline personality disorder. *Journal of Clinical Psychiatry, 48,* 15–22.

Degler, C. N. (1991). *In search of human nature.* Oxford, UK: Oxford University Press.

Denning, P. (1998). Therapeutic interventions for individuals with substance use, HIV, and personality disorders: Harm reduction as a unifying approach. *In Session: Psychotherapy in Practice, 4*(1), 37–52.

Dixon, L., Haas, G., & Weiden, P. (1990). Acute effects of drug abuse in schizophrenic patients: Clinical observations and patients' self-reports. *Schizophrenia Bulletin, 16*(1), 69–79.

Evans, K., & Sullivan, J. M. (1990). *Dual diagnosis: Counseling the mentally ill substance abuser.* New York: Guilford Press.

Fingarette, H. (1988). *Heavy drinking: The myth of alcoholism as a disease.* Berkeley: University of California Press.

Fox, V. (1993). *Addiction, change and choice.* Tucson, AZ: See Sharp Press.

Frances, R. J., & Miller, S. I. (Eds.). (1998). *Clinical textbook of addictive disorders* (2nd ed.). New York: Guilford Press.

Gabbard, G. O. (1992). Psychodynamic psychiatry in the "Decade of the Brain." *American Journal of Psychiatry, 149*(8), 991–997.

Gardner, E. (1997). Brain reward mechanisms. In J. Lowinson, P. Ruiz, R. Millman, & J. Langrod (Eds.), *Substance abuse: A comprehensive textbook* (pp. 51–84). Baltimore: Williams & Wilkins.

Gitlin, M. (1996). *The psychotherapist's guide to psychopharmacology* (2nd ed.). New York: Free Press.

Glantz, M., & Pickens, R. (Eds.). (1992). *Vulnerability to drug abuse.* Washington, DC: American Psychological Association.

Gordon, J., & Barrett, K. (1993). The codependency movement: Issues of context and differentiation. In J. Baer, A. Marlatt, & R. J. McMahon (Eds.), *Addictive behaviors across the life span: Prevention, treatment and policy issues* (pp. 307–339). Newbury Park, CA: Sage.

Gorman, M. (1994). *The etiology of addiction: A discussion of Joyce McDougall's theory of psychosomatic phenomena.* Unpublished manuscript, San Francisco School of Psychology.

Gorman, M. (1998). *Covert trauma, attachment theory, and addiction: A synthesis of theoretical and clinical implications.* Unpublished manuscript, San Francisco School of Psychology.

Grayer, E., & Sax, P. (1986). A model for the diagnostic and therapeutic use of countertransference. *Clinical Social Work Journal, 14*(4), 295–309.

Group for the Advancement of Psychiatry (D. Adler, Chairman, Committee on Psychopathology). (1987). *The Interactive fit: A guide to nonpsychotic chronic patients* (Report No. 121). New York: Brunner/Mazel.

Hasin, D. S., Tsai, W.-Y., Endicott, J., Mueller, T., Coryell, W., & Keller, M. (1996). The effects of major depression on alcoholism: Five-year course. *American Journal of Addictions, 5*(2), 144–155.

Herd, D. (1991). The paradox of temperance: Blacks and the alcohol question in nineteenth-century America. In S. Barrows & R. Room (Eds.), *Drinking: Behavior and belief in modern history* (pp. 254–375). Berkeley: University of California Press.

Hester, R. K., & Miller, W. R. (Eds.). (1989). *Handbook of alcoholism treatment approaches: Effective alternatives.* New York: Pergamon Press.

Horn, J. L., Wanberg, K. W., & Foster, F. M. (1987). *Guide to the Alcohol Use Inventory.* Minneapolis: National Computer Systems.

Horvath, A. T. (1998). *Sex, drugs, gambling, and chocolate: A workbook for overcoming addictions.* San Luis Obispo, CA: Impact.

Housner, R. (1993). Medication and transitional phenomena. In M. Schachter (Ed.), *Psychotherapy and medication* (pp. 87–108). Northvale, NJ: Aronson.

Inaba, D., Cohen, W., & Holstein, M. (1997). *Uppers, downers, all arounders* (3rd ed.). Ashland, OR: CNS Publications.

Insel, T. R. (1997). A neurobiological basis of social attachment. *American Journal of Psychiatry, 154*(6), 726–735.

Janis, I. L., & Mann, L. (1977). *Decision making.* New York: Free Press.

Kandel, D., & Davies, M. (1992). Progression to regular marijuana involvement: Phenomenology and risk factor for near-daily use. In M. Glantz & R. Pickens

(Eds.), *Vulnerability to drug abuse* (pp. 211–253). Washington, DC: American Psychological Association.

Kessler, R., Crum, R., Warner, L., & Nelson, C. (1997). Lifetime co-occurrence of DSM-III-R alcohol abuse and dependence with other psychiatric disorders in the National Comorbidity Study. *Archives of General Psychiatry, 54*(4), 313–321.

Kosten, T., & McCance, E. (1996). A review of pharmacotherapies for substance abuse. *American Journal on Addictions, 5*(4, Suppl. 1), 530–537.

Kranzler, H., & Anton, R. (1997). Implications of recent neuropsychopharmacologic research for understanding the etiology and development of alcoholism. In G. A. Marlatt & G. VandenBos (Eds.), *Addictive behaviors: Readings on etiology, prevention, and treatment* (pp. 68–93). Washington, DC: American Psychological Association.

Kroll, J. (1988). *The challenge of the borderline patient: Competency in diagnosis and treatment*. New York: Norton.

Krystal, H. (1988). *Integration and self-healing: Affect, trauma, and alexithymia*. Hillsdale, NJ: Analytic Press.

Krystal, H., & Raskin, H. (1970). *Drug dependence: The disturbances in personality functioning that create the need for drugs*. Northvale, NJ: Aronson.

Kuhn, C., Swartzwelder, S., & Wilson, W. (1998). *Buzzed: The straight facts about the most used and abused drugs from alcohol to ecstasy*. New York: Norton.

Leeds, J., & Morgenstern, J. (1996). Psychoanalytic theories of substance abuse. In F. Rotgers, D. S. Keller, & J. Morgenstern (Eds.), *Treating substance abuse: Theory and technique* (pp. 68–83). New York: Guilford Press.

Levin, J. (1991). *Treatment of alcoholism and other addictions: A self-psychology approach*. Northvale, NJ: Aronson.

Levin, J., & Weiss, R. (Eds.). (1994). *The dynamics and treatment of alcoholism: Essential papers*. Northvale, NJ: Aronson.

Little, J. G. (1999). *Introduction to harm reduction and motivational interviewing*. Lecture given at Department of Veterans Affairs Medical Center, San Francisco.

Little, J. G. (in press). Drop in groups: Harm reduction treatment for dually diagnosed adults. In A. Tatarsky (Ed.), *Varieties of success: A collection of stories about people who have successfully resolved problems with substance use*. Northvale, NJ: Aronson.

Manchester, W. (1992). *A world lit only by fire: The medieval mind and the Renaissance: Portrait of an age*. Boston: Back Bay Books.

Mark, D., & Faude, J. (1997). *Psychotherapy of cocaine addiction: Entering the interpersonal world of the cocaine addict*. Northvale, NJ: Aronson.

Marlatt, G. A. (1996). Harm reduction: Come as you are. *Addictive Behaviors, 21*, 779–788.

Marlatt, G. A. (Ed.). (1998a). *Harm reduction: Pragmatic strategies for managing high risk behaviors*. New York: Guilford Press.

Marlatt, G. A. (1998b). Horsing around at sobriety downs: A parable based on

Project MATCH [Special issue: Project MATCH]. *The Addictions Newsletter: The American Psychological Association, Division 50, 5*(2), 8–10.

Marlatt, G. A., & Gordon, J. (Eds.). (1985). *Relapse prevention: Maintenance strategies in the treatment of addictive behaviors.* New York: Guilford Press.

Marlatt, G. A., & Tapert, S. F. (1993). Harm reduction: Reducing the risks of addictive behaviors. In J. Baer, A. Marlatt, & R. J. McMahon (Eds.), *Addictive behaviors across the life span: Prevention, treatment and policy issues* (pp. 243–273). Newbury Park, CA: Sage.

McDougall, J. (1982). Alexithymia, a psychoanalytic viewpoint. *Psychotherapy Psychosomatics, 38,* 81–90.

McLellan, A. T., Luborsky, L., Woody, G., & O'Brien, C. (1980). An improved diagnostic evaluation instrument for substance abuse patients: The Addiction Severity Index. *Journal of Nervous and Mental Disease, 168,* 26–33.

McLellan, T., Alterman, A., Metzger, D., Grissom, G., Woody, G., Luborsky, L., & O'Brien, C. (1997). Similarity of outcome predictors across opiate, cocaine, and alcohol treatments: Role of treatment services. In G. Marlatt & G. VandenBos (Eds.), *Addictive behaviors: Readings on etiology, prevention, and treatment* (pp. 718–758). Washington, DC: American Psychological Association.

Medical Economics. (1998). *Physician's desk reference* (52 ed.). Montvale, NJ: Author.

Miller, W. R. (1976). Alcoholism scales and objective assessment methods: A review. *Psychological Bulletin, 83,* 649–674.

Miller, W. R. (1985). Motivation for treatment: A review with special emphasis on alcoholism. *Psychological Bulletin, 98,* 84–107.

Miller, W. R., & Hester, R. K. (1986). Inpatient alcoholism treatment: Who benefits? *American Psychologist, 41,* 794–805.

Miller, W., & Page, A. (1991). Warm turkey: Other routes to abstinence. *Journal of Substance Abuse Treatment, 8,* 227–232.

Miller, W. R., & Rollnick, S. (1991). *Motivational interviewing: Preparing people to change addictive behavior.* New York: Guilford Press.

Morgenstern, J., & Leeds, J. (1993). Contemporary psychoanalytic theories of substance abuse: A disorder in search of a paradigm. *Psychotherapy, 30,* 194–206.

Musto, D. F. (1987). *The American disease: Origins of narcotic control* (expanded ed.). New York: Oxford University Press.

Nash, M. (1997, May 5). Addicted. *Time,* pp. 69–76.

Nestler, E. (1995). Molecular basis of addictive states. *Neuroscientist, 1*(4), 212–219.

Nunes, E., Quitkin, F., Donovan, S., & Deliyannides, D. (1998). Imipramine treatment of opiate-dependent patients with depressive disorders: A placebo-controlled trial. *Archives of General Psychiatry, 55*(2), 153–160.

Ojehagen, A., & Berglund, M. (1989). Changes in drinking goals in a two-year outpatient alcoholic treatment program. *Addictive Behaviors, 14,* 1–9.

Pachman, J., Foy, D., & VanErd, M. (1978). Goal choice of alcoholics: A comparison of those who choose total abstinence vs. those who choose responsible, controlled drinking. *Journal of Clinical Psychology, 34,* 781–783.

Peele, S. (1991). *The truth about addiction and recovery.* New York: Simon & Schuster.

Prochaska, J., DiClemente, C., & Norcross, J. (1994). *Changing for good.* New York: Avon.

Prochaska, J., DiClemente, C., & Norcross, J. (1992). In search of how people change: Applications to addictive behaviors. *American Psychologist, 47*(9), 1102–1114.

Project MATCH Research Group. (1997). Matching alcoholism treatments to client heterogeneity: Project MATCH posttreatment drinking outcomes. *Journal of Studies on Alcohol, 58,* 7–29.

Regier, D., Farmer, M., & Rae, D. (1990). Comorbidity of mental disorders with alcohol and other drug abuse: Results from the epidemiologic catchment area (ECA) study. *Journal of the American Medical Association, 264*(19), 2511–2518.

Reinarman, C., & Levine, H. (1997). *Crack in America: Demon drugs and social justice.* Berkeley: University of California Press.

Ries, R., & Consensus Panel Chair. (1994). *Assessment and treatment of patients with coexisting mental and alcohol and other drug abuse* (Treatment Improvement Protocol Series No. 9). U.S. Department of Health and Human Services, Center for Substance Abuse Treatment, Publication No. [SMA] 94–2078.

Rotgers, F. (1998). The treatment of problem drinking using harm reduction techniques. In L. Vandecreek, S. Kuapp, & T. Jackson (Eds.), *Innovations in clinical practice: A sourcebook* (Vol. 16, pp. 65–79). Sarasota, FL: Professional Resource Press.

Sanchez-Craig, M., & Lei, H. (1986). Disadvantages of imposing the goal of abstinence on problems drinkers: An empirical study. *British Journal of Addiction, 81,* 505–512.

Saunders, J., & Aasland, O. (Eds.). (1987). *WHO collaborative project on identification and treatment of persons with harmful alcohol consumption: Report on phase I: Development of a screening instrument.* Geneva: World Health Organization.

Schore, A. (1994). *Affect regulation and the origin of the self.* Hillsdale, NJ: Erlbaum.

Schore, A. (1996). The experience-dependent maturation of a regulatory system in the orbital prefrontal cortex and the origin of developmental psychopathology. *Development and Psychopathology, 8,* 59–87.

Schuckit, M. (1989). *Drug and alcohol abuse: A guide to diagnosis and treatment* (3rd ed.). New York: Plenum.

Skinner, H. A., & Allen, B. A. (1983). Differential assessment of alcoholism. *Journal of Studies on Alcohol, 44,* 852–862.

Sobell, L. C., Cunningham, J. A., & Sobell, M. B. (1996). Recovery from alcohol problems with and without treatment: Prevalence in two population surveys. *American Journal of Public Health, 86,* 966–972.

Sobell, L. C., Cunningham, J. A., Sobell, M. B., & Toneatto, T. (1993). A Life-span perspective on natural recovery (self-change) from alcohol problems. In J. Baer, A. Marlatt, & R. J. McMahon (Eds.), *Addictive behaviors across the life span: Prevention, treatment and policy issues* (pp. 34–68). Newbury Park, CA: Sage.

Sobell, M. B., Sobell, L. C., Bogardis, J., Leo, G. I., & Skinner, W. (1992). Problem drinkers' perceptions of whether treatment goals should be self-selected or therapist-selected. *Behavior Therapy, 23,* 43–52.

Soloff, P. (1987). Neuroleptic treatment in the borderline patient: Advantages and techniques. *Journal of Clinical Psychiatry Supplement, 48,* 26–30.

Stahl, S. M. (1996). *Esssential psychopharmacology: Neuroscientific basis and practical applications.* New York: Cambridge University Press.

Springer, E. (1991). Effective AIDS prevention with active drug users: The harm reduction model. In M. Shernoff (Ed.), *Counseling chemically dependent people with HIV illness* (pp. 141–158). New York: Harrington Park Press.

Stimmel, B. (1997). *Pain and its relief without addiction: Clinical issues in the use of opioids and other analgesics.* New York: Haworth.

Substance Abuse and Mental Health Services Administration, Center for Substance Abuse Treatment. (1995). *Detoxification from alcohol and other drugs* (Treatment Improvement Protocol Series No. 19). Department of Health and Human Services, Rockville, MD.

Substance Abuse and Mental Health Services Administration. (1996, August). *Preliminary estimates from the 1995 national household survey on drug abuse* (Advance Report No. 18). Washington, DC: Office of Applied Studies.

Sullivan, H. S. (1954). *The psychiatric interview.* New York: Norton.

Tatarsky, A. (1998). An integrated approach to harm reduction psychotherapy: A case of problem drinking secondary to depression. *In Session: Psychotherapy in Practice, 4*(1), 9–24.

Thombs, D. L. (1994). *Introduction to addictive behaviors.* New York: Guilford Press.

Trimpey, J. (1992). *The small book* (rev. ed.). New York: Dell Trade Paperbacks.

Treece, C., & Khantzian, E. J. (1986). Psychodynamic factors in the development of drug dependence. *Psychiatric Clinics of North America, 9,* 399–412.

Tyrell, I. (1991). Women and temperance in international perspective: The world's Women's Christian Temperance Union. In S. Barrows & R. Room (Eds.), *Drinking: Behavior and belief in modern history* (pp. 217–242). Berkeley, CA: University of California Press.

van der Kolk, B. A. (1988). The trauma spectrum: The interaction of biological and social events in the genesis of the trauma response. *Journal of Traumatic Stress, 1*(3), 273–291.

van der Kolk, B. A., McFarlane, A. C., & Weisaeth, L. (Eds.). (1996). *Traumatic stress: The effects of overwhelming experience on mind, body, and society.* New York: Guilford Press.

Varma, S., & Siris, S. (1996). Alcohol abuse in Asian Americans: Epidemiological and treatment issues. *American Journal on Addictions, 5*(2), 136–143.

Volkow, N., Wang, G.-J., Fowler, J., Logan, J., Gatley, S., Gifford, A., Hitzemann, R., Ding, Y.-S., & Pappas, N. (1999). Prediction of reinforcing responses to psychostimulants in humans by brain dopamine D$_2$ receptor levels. *American Journal of Psychiatry, 156*(9), 1440–1443.

Walant, K. (1995). *Creating the capacity for attachment: Treating addictions and the alienated self.* Northvale, NJ: Aronson.

Weibel-Orlando, J. (1987). Culture-specific treatment modalities: Assessing client to treatment fit in Indian alcoholism programs. In M. Cox (Ed.), *Treatment and prevention of alcohol problems: A resource manual* (pp. 261–283). Orlando, FL: Academic Press.

Weil, A., & Rosen, W. (1993). *From chocolate to morphine.* Boston: Houghton Mifflin. (Original work published 1983)

Weiss, R., Najavits, L., Greenfield, S., & Soto, J. (1998). Validity of substance use self-reports in dually diagnosed outpatients. *American Journal of Psychiatry, 155*(1), 127–128.

Westermeyer, J. (1996). Alcoholism among new world peoples: A critique of history, methods, and findings. *American Journal of Addictions, 5*(2), 110–123.

Wurmser, L. (1978). *The hidden dimension: Psychodynamics of compulsive drug use.* New York: Aronson.

Yee, B. E. K., & Thu, N. D. (1987). Correlates of drug use and abuse among Indochinese refugees: Mental health implications. *Journal of Psychoactive Drugs, 19,* 77–83.

Zinberg, N. E. (1984). *Drug, set, and setting: The basis for controlled intoxicant use.* New Haven, CT: Yale University Press.

Zucker, E. (1995, October 21). *The practice of eclectic psychotherapy.* Presentation at the Russell Street Psychotherapy Institute symposium, Berkeley, CA.

Zweben, J., & Denning, P. (1998). *The alcohol and drug wildcard: Substance use and psychiatric problems in people with HIV* (UCSF AIDS Health Project Monograph Series No. 2.). San Francisco: UCSF AIDS Health Project.

# Author Index

247

# Subject Index

250